# Your Essential Guide To Understanding Sensory Processing Disorder

## BONUS SECTION!
Tips for Travelling with a Sensory Kiddo!

Written By: Angie Voss, OTR

Your Essential Guide to Understanding
Sensory Processing Disorder
Copyright © 2011 by Angie Voss, OTR
2nd Edition 2013
All Rights Reserved
**ISBN-13: 978-1466432642**

Dear Reader:

This handbook is also intended to be used with *Understanding Your Child's Sensory Signals* as well as **ASensoryLife.com**. Enjoy the BONUS section of "Travelling with a Sensory Kiddo"! My hope is that with all of these tools, you will develop an understanding of sensory processing which empowers you to be the voice for your child as well as the leader in living a life filled with sensory enrichment. Educating yourself is the first step. Your journey continues when you embrace and engage in living a sensory enriched life and most importantly, understanding and respecting your child's sensory differences.

All topics discussed in this guide are further addressed on **ASensoryLife.com**. I suggest using the search bar on the homepage to enter a keyword about which you would like to find more information. You will find printable handouts, sensory how-to videos, sensory tools and equipment ideas and links, and much, much more!

# Enjoy the Sensory Journey!

# Contents

Sensory 101 .................................................................................................. 6
    What is sensory processing disorder (SPD)? ................................................ 7
    What is sensory modulation? ...................................................................... 7
Sensory Over-Registration and Under-Registration .......................................... 8
    Over-Registration ...................................................................................... 8
        Tactile Over-Registration ..................................................................... 9
        Vestibular Over-Registration ............................................................. 11
        Auditory Over-Registration ............................................................... 12
    Under-Registration .................................................................................. 12
        Tactile Under-Registration ................................................................ 13
        Vestibular Under-Registration ........................................................... 13
        Proprioceptive Under-Registration .................................................... 14
The Power Sensations ................................................................................... 15
Oral Sensory Needs and Development ........................................................... 17
Proprioception, Proprioception, Proprioception! ............................................ 18
The Vestibular and Auditory Connection ....................................................... 21
The Power of Vestibular Input ....................................................................... 22
Self-Regulation and Ready State .................................................................... 24
    Sensory Anchors ...................................................................................... 26
    Fight or Flight ......................................................................................... 27
Sensory Meltdowns ....................................................................................... 29
Sensory or Behavior? .................................................................................... 30
S.E.N.S.E. © ................................................................................................. 31
More Bang for Your Sensory Buck! ................................................................ 32
The Survival Guide for Travelling with a Sensory Kiddo ................................ 34
    Why is Travelling so Difficult? ................................................................ 35
    Road Trip ................................................................................................ 36
    Airplanes ................................................................................................. 39
    Staying with Relatives or Friends ............................................................ 43

Hotels .................................................................................................................. 46

The Beach .......................................................................................................... 48

Camping and Hiking ......................................................................................... 50

Amusement Parks ............................................................................................. 52

Water Parks ....................................................................................................... 56

## Important Sensory Concepts

- Sensory kiddos do not realize they are experiencing sensation differently than someone else; therefore these children do not know how to express the sensation as being abnormal or different.
- Sensory stimuli can rule a sensory kiddo's life. It can be so powerful that it affects every move the child makes…craving it or avoiding it at all cost.
- If a baby or child cannot handle movement, it needs to be addressed and evaluated by a sensory integration OT. Movement (vestibular processing) is crucial for brain development and impacts development in many areas.
- Children naturally want to please others and do not intend to misbehave. All they really want is to be accepted and loved.
- Deep breathing is the quickest and most effective way to avoid fight or flight and triggering the sympathetic nervous system.
- The brain thrives on movement to attend and process information. Keep this in mind when it comes to learning and academics.
- A sensory kiddo may spend the entire day just trying to maintain ready state and self-regulate. This can be exhausting for the child.
- Before reacting with a reprimand or a punishment, consider a sensory tool or strategy.
- Sensory input is powerful, and understanding a child's sensory needs and differences can truly change the quality of life for that child.
- The brain responds best to purposeful and meaningful activities.
- Sensory needs and challenges can change on a day to day basis. One technique that may work one day may not be tolerated the next. This is the nature of SPD.

# Sensory 101

Contrary to popular belief, we have SEVEN senses, not five. These four are important, but not nearly as foundational as the 3 discussed below.

Visual (Sight)    Auditory (Sound)    Gustatory (Taste)    Olfactory (Smell)

The most important senses are frequently overlooked, and quite often not even recognized. And the thing is, they are critical for brain development and maturity! When we are talking about sensory integration and/or sensory processing (these two terms can be used interchangeably), the senses which impact sensory processing and development most powerfully are….

**Proprioception    Tactile    Vestibular**

### Proprioception
Proprioception is often referred to as "heavy/hard work" in the therapy world. Proprioceptive receptors are located in the joints, muscles, and tendons ALL OVER the body, including the jaw and vertebrae. These receptors are activated by elongation, compression, or traction; therefore, during heavy/hard work activities the core of the body and extremities recruit a large number of muscles. When the muscle bellies contract, the proprioceptors of the joints are triggered. Weight bearing on joints also triggers the proprioceptive receptors. The interoceptors are also a part of the proprioceptive system. They are located within the gut and internal organs. The interoceptors are responsible for the feeling of hunger or lack of hunger as well as the need to go to the restroom, and other internal organ sensations. Proprioception is tolerated very well by the nervous system and can be a tool for calming or alerting, depending on the need. The nervous system takes in the information and uses it accordingly. Proprioception is an excellent tool for calming, organizing, and self-regulating the nervous system. Fifteen minutes of a proprioceptive activity can have a 1-2 hour positive effect on sensory processing!

### Tactile
The tactile system involves the entire skin network including in the mouth, where tactile nerve endings are present in the cheek linings. Tactile input includes light touch, firm touch, and the discrimination of different textures including dry to wet and messy. The tactile system is also responsible for the processing of pain and temperature. Tactile input can be alerting, calming, or over-stimulating, depending on the person.

### Vestibular
When you think vestibular…think **movement and balance**. The vestibules are located in the inner ear and detect motion. There are 3 canals which detect different planes of movement. The various planes of movement all need to be processing correctly for a well-oiled machine. The planes of movement include:  1.) Back and forth; 2.) Side to side; 3.) Vertical, up and down; 4). Rotary; and 5.) Diagonal. Vertical input tends to be the most tolerated form of vestibular input, as well as the most regulating and organizing. Movement is crucial to development, not only perhaps the more obvious gross motor development and posture. Movement also plays a role in visual development, auditory processing, and overall self-regulation of the nervous system. Vestibular input is extremely powerful and can be alerting or calming to the nervous system. Vestibular development begins well

before a baby is born and while in utero the vestibular system is activated. Fifteen minutes of vestibular input can have a 6-8 hour positive (or negative) effect on the brain, depending on the person.

## What is sensory processing disorder (SPD)?

Sensory processing disorder is difficulty detecting, organizing, or responding to sensory information received and interpreted in the brain via all seven senses. We ALL have sensory processing differences; it can only be considered SPD when it causes significant difficulties in daily life, development, behavior, and social interactions. Sensory processing disorder is also sometimes called sensory integrative dysfunction, they means the same thing.

The three most common sensory systems affected with sensory processing disorder are **vestibular**, **proprioceptive**, and **tactile**. These three are also referred to as the power sensations and will be the primary focus of sensory based intervention as well as with a successful sensory home program.

Sensory differences and sensory processing disorder can present in different ways, and no two sensory kiddos are alike. A child may be a sensory avoider and over-register sensory information coming into the brain from one or more of the sensory systems. On the other hand, a child may be a sensory seeker, and under-register sensory information coming into the brain. A child may also present with a combination of the two types, in different sensory systems. And to complicate matters a little more, a child may have difficulty modulating the sensory input. This is often referred to as sensory modulation disorder.

## What is sensory modulation?

Sensory modulation is the process in which the brain is taking in all of the various types of sensory input and sorting it out and sending it to the right places in the brain. There is a specific place in the brain called the reticular activating system, which is like the hub and distribution center for the brain. The sensory information is then sorted out and sent out to the appropriate pathways for different aspects of daily function, self-regulation, ready state, etc.

My best analogy on this one is to think of the entrance to the brain for the sensory information as a conveyor belt, and the brain is all of the shelves for different organized items. So the boxes are coming in on the belt (sensory input) one after another and at the end of the belt (the reticular activating system) the boxes are being neatly sorted and put on the right shelves on a constant basis. So that is how the neuro-typical brain works.

**With our sensory kiddos, sensory modulation is often an issue, and the conveyor belt gets jammed up and piled up at the unloading spot. Or the conveyor belt is running REALLY slow and the shelves are quite empty. Sometimes it is as though the conveyor belt has a short in it, starting and stopping, starting and stopping.**

The tricky part is that this conveyor belt needs to be running at different speeds throughout the day such as waking up and getting going for the day, then maintaining ready state during the day, then transitioning back to a slower speed at night. And those with sensory modulation difficulties have a "conveyor belt" that is not real good at changing speeds at the right time.

# Sensory Over-Registration and Under-Registration

Sensory registration is how the brain processes and interprets incoming sensory input. Think of it like a computer...the keyboard being the incoming sensory message...the computer hard drive being the brain, which then interprets the input and completes a task. This is what sensory registration is all about. If this "hard drive" in the brain misinterprets sensory messages, it may miss the sensory information completely, over react to the input, or get overloaded to the point of a "crash" in the hard drive.

The neuro-typical brain is able to flow smoothly, interpreting and sorting out various sensory messages, and uses the relevant sensory input for an adaptive response to the environment. The child with sensory processing difficulties, unfortunately, is often unable to respond to the environment in an adaptive manner. This is observed through "output"... including delays in development and poor emotional control, behavior, social interaction, and maladaptive responses to the environment.

## Over-Registration

A brain that over-registers is unable to sort out the relevant from the irrelevant sensory stimuli and takes in every tiny sensory message. Too many sensory receptors are responding. This is also referred to as sensory defensiveness and can then be further classified based on the type, such as tactile defensiveness or auditory defensiveness. Some people in the therapy world may also call it over-responsivity. This type of child is often called a sensory avoider. I know this may be confusing at times, but all of these different words basically describe the same thing. In this workbook I will keep it simple with concepts of OVER and UNDER registration as a guide to understanding sensory signals.

Over-registration can occur with one type of sensory input such as tactile, or it may be multi-sensory, involving two or more senses such as visual, auditory, and vestibular. It can be any combination. Sensory stimuli, such as the feeling of clothing on our skin (tactile), are typically tuned out by the neuro-typical brain. A brain that over-registers tactile input may "feel" the clothes ALL day long, unable to adjust or habituate to the texture on the skin. This type of over-registration can happen with any of the senses, yet it is very unlikely to happen with proprioceptive input.

A child with sensory over-registration difficulties may present in different ways, although I will give some common characteristics.
- Easily distracted by sensory stimuli in their immediate environment
- Irritable or quick to melt down
- Frequent episodes of "fight or flight"
- On "high alert" at all times, appearing anxious
- Reserved, cautious around others
- Keeps to themselves
- Over-analyzes and approaches new activities and situations with extreme caution

Let's now break it down further to describe common characteristics or presentation of the most common sensory differences....

# Tactile Over-Registration
Also called: Tactile Defensiveness or Tactile Over-Responsivity

This is the child who often lashes out at others at school or in group settings. The child may be aggressive in nature because the nervous system is constantly feeling threatened by unexpected touch. Children are famous for getting into each other's personal bubble/space....therefore this can be extremely difficult for a child who perceives touch and texture as painful or noxious. This so called aggression or physically lashing out is actually a form of protection. Just as if you or I saw a bee flying right towards our eye, we would swat it away to protect ourselves, right? This is how children who over-register tactile input may react to others brushing against them, or a teacher lightly touching them or touching their hair in an endearing attempt to interact. The child may hold back from punching the teacher, but indeed will lash out and hit another child. The child is trying so hard to cope throughout the day at school that it may just take one seemingly harmless form of touch that sends the child through the roof and into complete sensory overload.
The presentation of tactile sensory overload comes in many forms...

- May just break down and cry and become inconsolable
- There may be a "fight or flight" reaction, possibly observed as trying to escape or flee from the current situation or lashing out by hitting, kicking, biting, etc.
- May try to hide somewhere . . . in a closet, under the table, under the sheets/blankets on the bed
- May try to self-protect by hiding behind someone, tucking in the arms and hands, covering the face or covering the skin by only wearing long pants and long-sleeved shirts, leaving a jacket on, or wanting to be wrapped in a blanket.

The tactile system is also responsible for regulating body temperature; therefore, a child who does not process tactile information efficiently may overheat easily or get cold easily. It is important to be aware of this when a child is outdoors. Watch for signs such as the child getting extremely red in the face, profuse sweating, or irritability. The child likely wants to keep playing and will not monitor this, so it is crucial to help the child by offering water or a shady cool down break. Be sure the child is not overdressed when it is hot out, and watch closely for a child who may get cold more quickly than others.

# The Connection between the Picky Eater and the Tactile System

There are tactile receptors located inside the mouth, in the linings of the cheeks and gums, and on the tongue. Of course eating is multi-sensory since taste and smell are also involved...but often the TEXTURE of the food is overlooked, which ties directly to over-registration of tactile input.

Be sure to respect this and honor the limitations, exploring textures via the mouth will naturally happen. You cannot force a child to just "get used to the texture". This must happen on its own, by offering various textured foods and also various textures in play. The tactile system will then learn to accept and process new tactile information. Actually forcing the issue can set the child back even further, as the nervous system will start to react in a "fight or flight" fashion instead of being open and accepting of new oral sensory experiences.

**Important Points to Consider in Regards to Tactile Over-Registration**
- Light touch can be very painful and unpleasant depending on the child.
- Deep pressure touch (firm touch) is very accepted by the body.
- Light touch can vary by the minute based on the state of regulation of the nervous system. One minute the child may like it and accept it, and the next minute it may send the child through the roof.
- Acceptance of touch is variable based on the state of the nervous system at any given moment for the child who over-registers tactile input.
- The response to tactile input can be unpredictable.
- When you first meet a child, you have no idea how the child processes tactile input, so ALWAYS stay in the safe zone and approach with firm pressure touch only. It is so common to see an adult/teacher/caregiver approach a child with light touch as a way of a gentle approach or caution, yet the approach actually should be the OPPOSITE.
- Just because a child is in a wheelchair, does not mean the child is fragile...the child would most likely love firm touch and a nice bear hug!
- Learning to approach others with firm touch in general is best.
- No wimpy, patting hugs! Give a nice firm pressure bear hug.
- Clothing is a HUGE issue for a child who over-registers tactile input! The designer jeans that the child was forced to wear because they were an expensive gift may cause pain and discomfort the ENTIRE day for the child. He/she will spend the whole day dealing with the sensation of the jeans! Let the child wear sweats or leggings if that is what is desired!
- The tactile system is responsible for regulation of temperature.
- A kiddo may appear to be shy or timid, but may not be at all...the child may just be protecting the tactile system.

# Vestibular Over-Registration
Also called: Vestibular Defensiveness or Vestibular Over-Responsivity

The vestibular system is very complex and responsible for SO many aspects of development, including self-regulation and the developmental milestones of rolling, crawling, and walking. It also plays a big role in posture and muscle tone. Gross motor coordination and auditory processing are directly linked to vestibular processing.

A child who over-registers vestibular input may not be able to tolerate movement in all planes or perhaps may tolerate it in just one plane. The different planes of movement are: side to side, back and forth, vertical (bouncing, jumping), rotary, and various diagonal planes which are not linear and are combinations of the linear planes. It is indeed possible that children LOVE swinging side to side, yet get nauseated going back and forth.

The presentation of vestibular over-registration can be observed in different ways...
- May avoid movement completely, including walking down a gentle slope; fearful of running or jumping
- May self-protect very well by having elaborate excuses and reasons as to why he/she "doesn't like to swing or slide"
- Often delays in gross motor skills
- Trying new things involving movement often avoided
- Prefers sedentary activities and may excel at fine motor tasks
- Even 30 seconds of swinging or movement in a plane of movement may not be tolerated well, and may cause a systemic reaction such as nausea, flushing of the skin, irritability, or a fight or flight response.
- May be fearful of the feet leaving the ground at all. The clinical term for this is "gravitational insecurity".

**Important Points to Consider in Regards to Vestibular Over-Registration**
- Respect the signs of vestibular distress. STOP means STOP.
- A child needs to know that you can be trusted and that you will honor the need to stop a new movement activity.
- Even one minute of vestibular input can be beneficial to sensory processing. More is not necessarily better unless the child's nervous system is ready.
- On the other hand, even one minute too much of vestibular input can cause hours of dysregulation for the child.
- Fifteen minutes of vestibular input can have a 6-8 hour effect on the brain, positive or negative, depending on how the brain processed the information.
- Vestibular input can be calming or alerting depending on the speed, duration, and intensity of the movement.
- A child may be swinging and appearing to enjoy it, and at any given moment may need to stop due to the powerful input to the brain.

## Auditory Over-Registration
Also called: Auditory Defensiveness or Auditory Over-Responsivity

Auditory input comes in various frequencies and tones. Quick changes in tone and the pitch and speed of sound can also vary. A child can over-register one frequency or tone and process another in a typical fashion. This is why some sounds bother a child and not others. Auditory input can be very painful and uncomfortable for a child, causing dysregulation or a fight or flight response. This over-registration of the auditory input can also cause a child to have a difficult time sorting out the irrelevant sounds in the environment, such as the sound of the refrigerator or the sound of the heater in the classroom. The child tapping a pencil or foot can be incredibly difficult to tune out for the child who over-registers auditory input. The other factor is unexpected loud sounds....for a child who over-registers this is very likely to cause a fight or flight reaction.

The presentation of auditory over-registration can be observed in different ways...
- Easily startled and frightened
- Covers the ears in expectation of loud sounds or as a reaction to sound
- Episodes of fight or flight often observed in chaotic environments or places where noises are very loud and unexpected (movie theater, gymnasium, parade, etc)
- May avoid group situations, ask to leave a party, or move away from guests in the home
- Very easily distracted and may have difficulty staying on task
- Often asks others to repeat something and has difficulty processing what was heard

## Under-Registration

Under-registration of sensory input is the exact opposite of over-registration. As the sensory information is coming into the brain and being processed, the information is getting lost, misinterpreted, or shuffled. It is as if you are hitting the keys on the keyboard for the computer, and the letters are just not popping up on the screen.

Sensory input is CRUCIAL for development, self-regulation, mood, behavior, emotions, social interaction, and language. The most important senses are tactile, vestibular, and proprioception when it comes to the impact on the brain; therefore, if a child is under-registering sensory information, it affects life in every aspect.

Under-registration can occur with one type of sensory input such as tactile, or it may be multi-sensory, involving two or more senses such as proprioception, auditory, and vestibular. It can be any combination.

A child with sensory under-registration difficulties may present in different ways, although I will give some common characteristics:
- Pre-occupied by sensation in the environment, as though they are sensory starved
- Irritable or quick to melt down
- On the move, constantly seeking movement, proprioception, and/or tactile input
- Quick changes in mood

- Difficulty with sleep patterns: falling asleep, staying asleep, waking up
- Difficulty staying on task and maintaining attention for sit down tasks
- Often clumsy, poor posture, difficulty with motor skills, low muscle tone
- Seeks out spicy and sour foods
- Unable to determine body in space, has difficulty with body awareness
- Is a thrill seeker...would jump off the roof if allowed
- Delays in speech and language development
- Difficulty with motor planning

Let's now break it down further to describe common characteristics or presentation of the most common sensory differences for under-registration....

## Tactile Under-Registration

Also called: Tactile Seeker or Tactile Under-Responsivity

Imagine if you could not FEEL things such as the soft texture of puppy or the feeling of the sand in between your toes on the beach. If so, you would likely seek out tactile input constantly right? This is what you may see with a tactile seeker. This under-registration of tactile information also impacts tactile discrimination, body awareness, and stereognosis. As previously mentioned, pain and temperature are also controlled by the tactile system.

The presentation of tactile under-registration comes in different forms...

- Tends to touch everything, including other people's skin, hair, clothing, etc.
- Constantly fidgeting with something in the hands while trying to attend or learn
- Cannot get enough of textures (wants to roll around in the sandbox)
- LOVES messy play
- Does not respond to extreme temperatures like others
- Lacks body awareness, physical boundaries, and body in space awareness
- May not feel pain like others; e.g., may get burned and not even react . . . this type of child usually does not mind shots at the doctor's office!

## Vestibular Under-Registration

Also called: Vestibular Seeker or Vestibular Under-Responsivity

Vestibular input plays an enormous role in motor development, posture, kinesthesia, ocular control, auditory processing (yep, auditory) and self-regulation. Imagine swinging and not feeling the motion or spinning and not getting dizzy. Childhood is about moving and grooving and playing your little heart out! There indeed is a reason for this...the brain thrives on MOVEMENT for development. We need it, and when a brain is starved of the sensation of movement, it will naturally seek it out.

The presentation of vestibular under-registration comes in different forms...
- Wants to swing, bounce, slide for hours on end
- The bigger the push on the swing and the higher the slide, the better
- Spins and spins and does not get dizzy
- Difficulty attending to tasks, especially when seated
- Constantly moving and changing position in a chair
- Never just walks...runs, hops, skips, jumps, etc.
- Difficulty with gross motor skills

## Proprioceptive Under-Registration

Also called: Proprioceptive Seeker

Proprioception, in my sensory experience opinion, is the most important sense of all . . . so important that I have written an entire chapter about it. If you noticed, I did not include proprioception in the over-registration section, which was not a mistake. The brain is not likely to over-register proprioception nor get over-stimulated by it. But the very unfortunate part is that it is very common for sensory kiddos to under-register proprioception. This can impact many areas of development and greatly impact self-regulation. The brain thrives on proprioception in so many ways, so when a child does not register this information it can cause many difficulties for the child.

The presentation of proprioceptive under-registration comes in many different forms...
- Poor posture, lacks body awareness and body in space
- Lacks coordination, appears clumsy, and shows delay in gross and fine motor skill.
- Difficulty with speech
- Poor muscle tone of mouth (drooler)
- Leans on everything and/or rubs body along surfaces
- Difficulty with sleep
- Emotional instability
- Difficulty attending to tasks, easily distracted
- Unpredictable change in mood
- Loves tight spaces and big bear hugs
- Does not recognize a personal bubble
- Preoccupied by sensation
- Frequent meltdowns

# The Power Sensations
## Proprioception  Vestibular  Tactile

Proprioceptive, vestibular, and tactile input are called the "power sensations" due to the fact that they are the foundation for sensory integration and sensory processing skills. These three types of input provide the basis for brain development (besides the autonomic functions of the nervous system such as respirations and heart rate).

When you work on one area, it impacts the processing of the other two in many ways. The complex processing of the brain and the pathways in which these three sensations integrate is the **key to success**!

Now here's the thing...almost all children with sensory processing challenges have difficulty processing information in at least one of these three areas, **often all three**.

The power sensations are the foundation and root of all development. Incorporating sensory activities from these three categories is essential for all children. And for those children who have sensory processing difficulties, it is critical. This may sound like a daunting task, but it doesn't have to be! When you live a sensory life and set up your home as a sensory friendly environment, it becomes a part of your child's day in a meaningful and purposeful way!

**Think of your child as a tree. The roots must be healthy, strong, and well fed in order for the tree to even begin to grow. Only then does the trunk of the tree begin to develop. Then some branches will grow, and eventually the leaves. And over time with adequate water, rich soil with all of the necessary nutrients, and sunshine (compare to a sensory enriched life)...only then will you find a lush, green, strong, and mature tree. This is the EXACT concept behind sensory integration. You wouldn't just water a leaf on a tree and expect it to grow and thrive, would you? You wouldn't just sprinkle a branch with dirt to give it nutrition and expect for leaves to grow, would you? Provide a sensory enriched life for your child, focusing on the power sensations, and watch your little tree grow.**

# Getting to the "Root" of Development

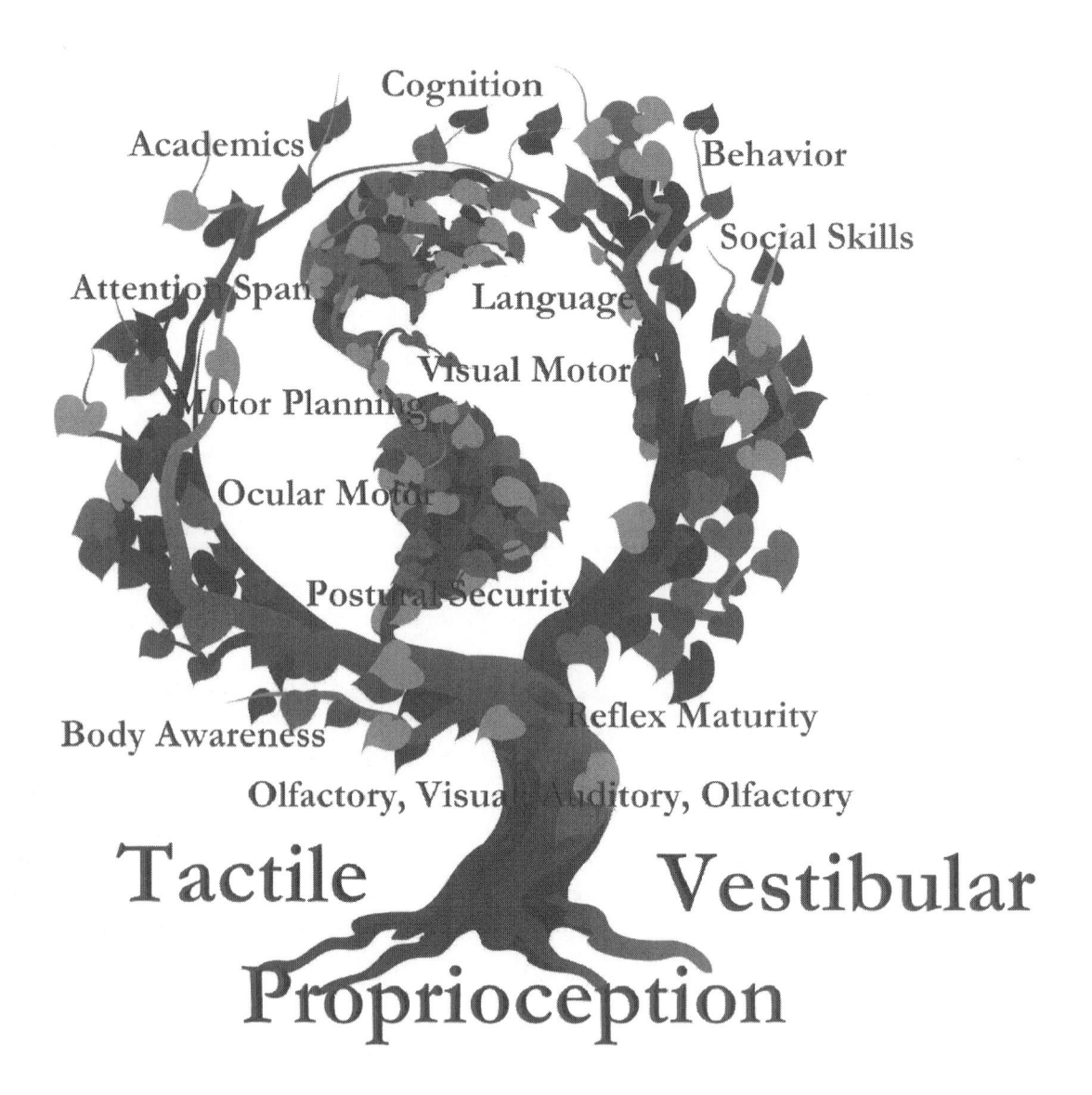

Cognition
Academics
Behavior
Social Skills
Attention Span
Language
Visual Motor
Motor Planning
Ocular Motor
Postural Security
Body Awareness
Reflex Maturity
Olfactory, Visual, Auditory, Olfactory

# Tactile     Vestibular
# Proprioception

# Oral Sensory Needs and Development
### A crucial and primitive link

Beginning in fetal development, oral sensory needs are evident, and these oral sensory needs are observed through the developmental stages as well as for self-regulation throughout our lives as children and adults. The types of sensory input received orally are complex and various....from basic suck/swallow/breath patterns of respiration, to the proprioception received through biting, chewing, and sucking provided to the jaw joints and the muscles of the tongue and cheeks. Additional sensory input is also received through the tactile receptors in the mouth for texture. The final sensory systems involved are taste and smell. With all of this said...it is pretty clear as to why we see our sensory kids with so many oral sensory differences....from oral aversion and being picky eaters, to those who want to chew and lick everything! Oral sensory input is often crucial for self-regulation and maintaining a ready state of arousal for these sensory kids. Something as simple as providing an oral sensory tool, encouraging deep breaths, or a resistive blowing activity can have a significant impact on self-regulation, mood, behavior, and attention to task. So, most importantly, allow the child to chew on something if needed. Do not treat it as a behavior, because it is not. Children who bite themselves or others is likely seeking oral sensory input to help self-regulate, and not trying to hurt someone. Providing the child with the appropriate oral tool and strategy is how you can help.

### Oral Sensory Activities and Tools

- Provide ongoing/available access to some sort of chewy. There are many commercially available chewy tools. It is important that it is somehow attached to the child, either by a clip or bracelet (necklace not recommended for safety for young children). My favorite is the Ark's Grabber® and it comes in different flavors, such as grape, chocolate, lemon, vanilla. Using a CamelBak® water bottle is also a great way to have an available chewy, as the mouthpiece provides excellent oral sensory feedback as well as resistive sucking. Kid Companions makes a variety of safe necklaces with a chewy pendant. They are great for all ages and do not stand out as a "therapy tool".
- Eating crunchy or chewy foods is also an effective way to provide needed oral sensory input. Suggestions: turkey jerky, fruit leather, bagels, pretzels, nuts, carrot sticks, crushed ice.
- Use small straws, such as coffee stirrers, or regular straws to drink smoothies, yogurt, or pudding to provide resistive sucking input.
- Provide chewing gum, especially the "real" chewing gum like Big League Chew® or Hubba Bubba®.
- Encourage the use of mouth toys such as a harmonica, whistle, kazoo, recorder, etc.
- One of my favorite activities and a sensory kiddo's favorite is blowing a "bubble mountain"! Using a long piece of Theratubing® or aquarium tubing as the straw....fill a large bowl or pitcher half way with water and add dish soap. Then have the child use the tube to blow the bubble mountain! It creates resistance with the blowing and encourages deep breaths which help tremendously with self-regulation. HINT: Be sure to "test the waters" before adding soap to make sure the child can coordinate blowing only.

# Proprioception, Proprioception, Proprioception!

Proprioception is the key to treatment for PT, OT, and SLP sessions! It is also the key to success in the classroom, and at home. I can't stress enough how effective proprioceptive input can be for the nervous system and sensory processing.

Probably the biggest reason proprioceptive input is the best thing since sliced gluten free bread is that you can't get too much of it! It is very accepted by all nervous systems, and there are TONS of ways to get it without the use of equipment or special training . . . and kids LOVE it!

Proprioception should be part of every single treatment in the clinic. I also suggest incorporating proprioception at home and school in doses throughout the day. A "dose" can be something as simple as wheelbarrow walking from one room to another or bear crawling as a transition to the next activity at school.

### Deep Pressure Touch (Activates Proprioceptive and Tactile Systems)

Deep pressure touch, also called hand hugs or squeezes, is an excellent staple to have in your sensory bag of tricks. It is extremely organizing and regulating for the brain. It provides firm pressure touch (tactile) as well as proprioceptive input. Deep pressure touch can be done to the arms, legs, feet, hands, head, cheeks, back…just avoid the chest and abdomen. It can be done in short intervals, even when you are just walking by the child and stop for a little dose of deep pressure touch. Or, it can take 10-15 minutes as an activity to help a child through a meltdown or at bedtime to help the child fall asleep. Let the child be your gauge. This is a valuable tool for parents since it can be done anywhere and doesn't require any special sensory equipment besides the hands.

### Heavy/Hard Work

In the sensory world you will often hear proprioception and heavy/hard work used interchangeably. This is because all heavy/hard work activates the proprioceptive system. Any activity that engages the muscles and requires muscle recruitment provides proprioceptive input. Postural engaging and core strength activities also involve proprioception. It is not necessary to have a child move a couch across the room to be considered heavy/hard work.

### Beyond the Ankles

A little bird told me one day that some therapists are often taught in school that proprioception only involves the ankles. Proprioceptors are actually all over the body, in every single muscle and joint, even the jaw and vertebrae! But back to the ankles…I want to discuss toe walking for a moment. Toe walking is often very misunderstood. Some consider it behavior, and sometimes it is mistaken for a tactile issue. BUT, it is likely more related to self-regulation when toe walking is discovered by the child to "feel good" and help them feel calm. The brain then remembers it as a calming tool, and it becomes something the child does all of the time. It is indeed important to assess the range of motion (ROM) in the ankles to be sure the tendon has not shortened. But if full ROM is still present, let the child do it! Toe walking is not disruptive, and it is not harmful to the child…but for some reason our society has decided it is not ok.

## Joint Traction

Joint traction is a form of proprioception. It occurs when there is tension, pull, or traction placed on a joint. It is very important for developing body awareness and body in space. It also promotes self-regulation and can be very calming, regulating, and organizing for the brain and nervous system.

**Natural Ways to Achieve Joint Traction:**
- Climb or hang from a tree
- Hang from a bar at the playground, on a trapeze bar, chin up bar, or railing
- Hang from knees hooked over a playground bar or trapeze bar
- Drape backwards over a large therapy ball, arms over head
- Hang over the side of the bed
- Stretching activities or yoga
- Theraband® activities
- Heavy/hard work activities involving pulling things such as a wagon
- Carry heavy objects such as a water pail

## Joint Compression

Joint compression is also a form of proprioception. It is the exact opposite of joint traction and occurs when there is compression, push, or weight bearing placed on a joint. It is essential for developing body awareness and body in space, as well as for joint stability and strength. Joint compression also promotes self-regulation and can be very calming, regulating, and organizing for the brain and nervous system.

**Natural Ways to Achieve Joint Compression:**
- Any weight bearing activity such as jumping, running, hopping, skipping
- Wheelbarrow walking
- Yoga poses
- Theraband® activities
- Trampoline, BOSU® ball, or hippity hop ball
- Hand stands or cartwheels
- Pogo stick
- Bike riding
- Heavy/hard work activities involving pushing such as a shopping cart or heavy box
- Crab walking
- Climbing activities at the playground (climb slides)
- Climbing hills

## Head/Neck Compression

A head/neck compression is also a form of joint compression that is achieved through downward pressure to the top of the head, compressing the vertebrae of the spine in the neck area. This can be very regulating and calming for the nervous system. Not only is the compression beneficial to the nervous system, but it also quite often involves inverting the head, which is that much more bang for your sensory buck!

**Natural Ways to Achieve Head/Neck Compression:**
- Head stands or other postures where head is compressed on the floor
- Drape over a large therapy ball with head on the floor (be sure to stabilize the ball for the child)

- In crawling position, push head firmly into a soft object such as a beanbag or pillow cave
- Have the child stand in a body sock with the sock pulled over the head

**More ideas for incorporating <u>proprioception</u> into the day!**
- Wheelbarrow walking
- Carry heavy items (laundry basket with clothes, groceries)
- Chewing gum or resistive chewy foods such as jerky or thick sourdough bread
- Drinking thick food through a straw (milkshakes, smoothies, yogurt, pudding, applesauce)
- Push or pull heavy items; wagon full of heavy stuff or maybe a sibling
- Dig in the dirt or sandbox with a shovel
- Play games with the cushions from the couch….squish under them, jump on them, crash into them, play sandwich games with them
- Pull siblings or friends around on a sheet or blanket
- Rollerblade, bike
- Rake leaves, shovel snow
- Push a wheelbarrow
- Carry buckets of water around outside
- Pillow fights
- Deep pressure hugs, bear hugs
- Use heavy quilts for bedding and tight pajamas
- Heavy weighted blankets, weighted lap pad
- Compression clothing such as Under Armour® athletic clothes, leotards, lifejacket, tight leggings
- Swimming
- Gymnastics
- Vacuum, wash the car
- Make a pillow cave in a duvet or small tent
- Climbing activities (climb a hill, climb a tree)
- Climb up slides
- Hang from a trapeze bar or stationary bar
- Headstands against the wall
- Activities on a large therapy ball: roll on it and walk on hands, lie over backwards and gently rock back and forth from hands to feet, roll therapy ball firmly over the child while he/she lies on stomach on the floor
- Pogo stick, hippity hop ball
- Burrito roll up: roll up the child tightly in a blanket (with head exposed)
- Crab walking, bear walking, leap frog
- Trampoline or BOSU® ball
- Weighted backpack
- Vibrating pillow or toy. (Never let the child place in ears. Also, if the child has a seizure disorder, it is important to consult with your OT prior to this activity.)
- Squish box (a storage box just the right size for your kiddo to squeeze into with pillows)
- Marching, stomping, skipping, running, hopping
- Play catch with a heavy/weighted ball
- Crawl through fabric tunnel, push large items through the tunnel
- Wrestling, gentle rough-housing

# The Vestibular and Auditory Connection

The vestibular and auditory systems have a very unique sensory connection. They share a cranial nerve that sends input to the brain. This is the vestibulocochlear nerve. Although it is not necessary to remember the name of this nerve, the shared connection is extremely important to understand due to the impact on sensory processing. Basically when the brain is receiving auditory input, the vestibular system is being activated, and vice versa. Soooooooooo . . . incorporating the two in therapy or at play is powerful because when one is activated the other is ready to rumble!

**When a child is engaged in a movement activity…. involve listening and auditory processing skills. Here are some ideas:**

- Play a listening game
- Sing songs
- Play soft instrumental music in background
- Use a metronome and follow the beat by clapping hands or using a musical instrument
- Play memory or guessing games
- Play category games

**When a child is engaged in an auditory learning activity….involve movement.**
This applies especially to speech and language therapy sessions and in the classroom at school OR during schoolwork done at home. Do you ever wonder why some children have a difficulty sitting still during a sit down learning activity? Well, their little brains are trying so hard to process the auditory information and make sense out of it. The brain knows that the vestibular system can help them! Therefore, you will see the child trying to "get vestibular input" via fidgeting in the seat, trying to stand up, bounce in the chair, etc. The brain thrives on movement to learn, attend, and process information. It is unfortunate that our society and educational system has decided that sitting still is the best way to learn.

But there is hope! More and more schools are being educated in regards to sensory needs! Ball chairs and T-stools are sometimes being used in the classrooms instead of regular school chairs. Simply sitting on a ball chair or T-stool activates the vestibular system. You don't have to be bouncing across the room to activate the vestibular system. Give it a try! Replace your office chair with a large therapy ball! I bet you will love it.

**Let's talk a little bit more about the vestibular system…**

# The Power of Vestibular Input

I will not go into the technical details of the vestibules and how all of the canals work. What I would like to go over is the **enormous impact** that the vestibular system has on sensory integration and self-regulation. (Refer back to the tree diagram.)

Movement is critical for brain development beginning in utero. Then after birth, it is how we calm infants and also how we make them smile and giggle. We rock them, bounce them, swing them, and sway them. All of this movement is doing a whole lot more than putting them to sleep or making us smile. It is creating a foundation for the brain and development. This need for movement continues throughout life and is especially crucial in the developmental years of childhood.

BUT…here's the thing…our society is evolving to be more and more sedentary by the minute. Every type of screen imaginable is out there. Television, computer, phones, hand held gaming devices, screens in the car, DVDs and movies in the schools, etc. AND our children our watching these screens even as infants! Research shows that the average child gets 6-8 hours of screen time a DAY! The bottom line is…this is a real problem. I don't know how else to put it.

Children are no longer outside climbing trees, playing in the mud, playing a game of four square, or even riding their bikes. But as you might guess…this is EXACTLY what our brains need to develop and promote self-regulation.

### Key Points on Vestibular Input and How to Make a Difference

- Every child should have an opportunity to get up and move every 15 minutes. Even just a quick stretch is beneficial.

- Inverting the head is very powerful and an excellent tool for a quick dose of vestibular input.

- Fifteen minutes of swinging can have a 6-8 hour effect on the brain.

- Remember the various planes of movement, and be sure to incorporate all of them; but allow rotary input only in controlled doses.

- Vertical vestibular input (bouncing and jumping) is typically the most accepted form of vestibular input and is very regulating and organizing since it involves a great deal of proprioception.

- Whenever possible, offer options besides sitting in a chair…lying on the floor propped on elbows, standing on a balance board, standing on a BOSU® ball, sitting on a ball chair or T-stool, etc.

- Discourage spinning! This can be very disorganizing for the brain and can cause delayed sensory overload. Monitor spinning to one revolution per second and a maximum of ten revolutions, then switch directions.

- Respect a child's reaction to vestibular input as it can be very powerful and have a systemic effect. Stop means stop if the child has had enough. Watch closely for signs of sensory overload if the child is unable to verbally communicate.

**More ideas for incorporating <u>vestibular</u> input into the day!**
- Jumping, hopping, skipping, running
- Rolling across the floor
- Tumbling and gymnastics
- Bike riding
- Scooter board
- Scooter or skateboard
- Rollerblading
- Pogo stick
- Swinging, indoors and outdoors
- Slides
- Jumping on the bed
- Hippity hop ball
- BOSU® ball
- Mini-trampoline or outdoor trampoline
- Therapy ball activities
- Dancing
- Yoga
- Rolling down hills

# Self-Regulation and Ready State

Self-regulation is the ability to adjust or regulate the level of alertness depending on the time of the day and the stimuli presented. For instance, the ability to wake up in the morning, become alert and adapt to the school environment and demands placed on the nervous system in the school setting…including attention to task, cognitive demands, communication, social and emotional demands, and motor tasks (gross, fine, and visual motor). Then returning home for the evening and preparing the nervous system for rest and sleep. The ability to self-regulate the nervous system involves all of these components, including the sleep/wake cycle. Children with sensory differences quite often have a difficult time with self-regulation due to various factors. Adapting to the environment and constantly changing needs and demands on the nervous system requires very complex processing in the brain, which is often taken for granted. When children have difficulty with self-regulation, maladaptive behavior or responses to the environment and sensory stimuli may be observed. It is very important to identify these signals of self-regulation before jumping to conclusion that it is behaviorally driven. Depending on the neurobehavioral state of the brain, the child may need an increased amount of sensory input or a decreased amount of sensory input.

Ready state is the state or level in which the brain and nervous system are ready to learn, adapt, adjust, transition, and take in sensory input. The computer analogy may also be applied here. When you turn a computer on, it needs time to warm up and gather all of the necessary information to then have a display screen that is ready for use. Sometimes the computer needs to be "re-booted" and sometimes it "crashes". These are all similar to how the brain works in its ability to process sensory information. Our sensory kiddos tend to have quite a few more crashes and re-boots. Their brains often need to warm up longer or possibly have more frequent warm-ups throughout the day if their "computer" (brain) was not in an active state of learning.

**Ready State**
- Engages and responds
- Catches on, "gets it"
- Keeps up with the flow of events
- Adapts to situational changes
- Stays busy with tasks that are meaningful
- Able to engage in challenging activities
- Interacts freely, initiates and participates
- Can be spontaneous and flexible
- Unexpected events are easily accepted
- Feels safe, comfortable, free of confusion
- Looks at ease, content
- Relaxed, but alert and attentive
- Not overwhelmed
- Confident in trying something new

**Not Ready State**
- Brain is preoccupied with sensation
- Difficulty with transitions
- Needs predictability
- Needs to be in control
- May appear upset
- Fearful or anxious
- Reacting to all sensory stimuli
- Easily overwhelmed
- Preoccupied with safety
- Explosive behavior
- Unable to attend to task
- Lethargic or always sleepy

## Dysregulation...Co-Regulation...Self-Regulation

There is a process in which the brain learns and develops the ability to self-regulate. For our sensory kiddos, this process can be much more difficult, and the amount of time spent dysregulated is greater than the neuro-typical brain. We are taught to help children self-regulate by providing the necessary sensory tools, and we expect them to do so independently. This is strongly recommended and very essential, **BUT sometimes the most important step is missed . . . co-regulation.**

Co-regulation is when a person feeds off of the state of regulation of those around them. And our sensory kiddos are like regulating sponges! They sense it all and they feel the stress of others. The child can also sense frustration, disappointment, sadness, and is extremely sensitive to the state of regulation of those around them. This includes if and when a parent or teacher is stressed, anxious, unsettled, angry, or irritated (even when it is not directly related to that child). This can also include your tone of voice, speed of talking, pitch in your voice, and body language. Even too much excitement and praise can be overwhelming and create a state of sensory overload...so be aware of this end of things, as well. A sensory kiddo does NOT do well in a rushed, intense, loud, multi-sensory environment...even the sensory seekers. Occasionally this is fine, and completely part of life...but not on a day to day basis. Remember that the child is co-regulating from those around him minute by minute.

Sensory kiddos rely on those around them to help "co-anchor and co-regulate" and to help achieve and maintain a state of self-regulation. Think of it this way...let's say you are outside in a horrible wind storm, 100mph winds, and the stop sign at the corner is the only thing for you to hang on to keep you safe and from blowing away. **Well, this could be how our children with SPD may feel...like their world and life is a constant "wind storm"...and YOU are the stop sign. The wind storm is dysregulation and the stop sign is co-regulation.** It is SO important for us as parents to be that solid rock, a stable and calm co-anchor and co-regulator in all situations. Our sensory kiddos may already see this world as a scary, unpredictable, out of sorts, and sometimes painful kind of place...we need to be that safe place and solid rock they can rely on in challenging and stressful situations and moments.

**Key Points in Helping Achieve Self-Regulation and Ready State**
- Proprioception is HUGE in regards to its impact on self-regulation and ready state. Proprioceptive activities are your "go to" sensory activities to help warm up or calm down the nervous system. The brain will respond accordingly.
- Compression clothing is an excellent tool for providing doses of proprioception throughout the day, therefore assisting in self-regulation and maintaining ready state.
- Hand flapping, toe walking, chewing on things, pulling on hair, and hanging onto an adult are some examples of a child trying to self-regulate and achieve ready state.
- Providing a sensory retreat for use throughout the day is crucial at home, in the clinic, and at school to help a child regulate and maintain ready state.
- Watch your voice level, speed of talking, and pitch…these can all affect a child's state of self-regulation.
- Vestibular input is effective for achieving ready state, as it can be calming or alerting.
- Deep breathing is an excellent tool to use throughout the day to assist in self-regulation.
- Resistive sucking or blowing activities, such as the bubble mountain, are also very effective.

## Sensory Anchors

A sensory anchor is a behavior or quite often a repetitive activity that helps the brain feel "good". It is a sensory signal indicating the child is feeling dysregulated or is in need of a dose of an organizing, calming sensation. For our sensory kiddos, the world can be a scary, unpredictable, disorganizing, and often uncomfortable place to be. When our children discover a sensory based activity that feels good to them, they tend to do it over and over. We all do this in some fashion! A sensory anchor helps the child feel grounded and in control of the moment, thereby achieving a sense of brain organization and regulation. It is very common to see an increase in sensory anchoring when the child is tired, stressed, challenged, or in a new multi-sensory situation. Here are some examples of possible sensory anchors.....

- Lining up toys/objects
- Following a line or straight surface with the eyes
- Staring at a spinning object
- Hand flapping
- Toe walking
- Making repetitive mouth sounds
- Chewing on things
- Smelling objects or a new environment/room

It is very important to respect these sensory signals and let the child do it! I do realize that some children perseverate and become fixated on a sensory anchor...and this is when you come into play! Encourage and transition to a FUN heavy/hard work play activity, movement activity, or tactile activity which will also help the brain regulate and feel good! The bubble mountain is a great choice as well! Also, be sure to give a warning that it will be time to move on to something else if the child becomes stuck in the sensory anchor activity.

# Fight or Flight

Research shows that children with Sensory Processing Disorder and sensory processing differences have a greater tendency to switch from the PNS (parasympathetic nervous system) to the SNS (sympathetic nervous system) based on adverse stimuli or an environment with new or a great amount of sensory stimuli.

**Parasympathetic nervous system**: This is where our nervous system remains most of the time and where we demonstrate a "ready state" for learning, social interaction, and just being alert and awake.

**Sympathetic nervous system**: The state of "fight or flight". This part of our nervous system is intended for safety and the ability to react in a dangerous situation.

Understanding what fight or flight looks like with a child is CRUCIAL in determining how to respond. The primitive and actual purpose of fight or flight is to divert blood from the brain to the muscles in order to respond quickly and with great strength as needed. For instance, you hear stories about the mom who lifted the car or tree off of her child...the mom was obviously in fight or flight to protect her child and the brain and nervous system responded accordingly. When the blood is diverted to the muscles instead of the brain, the brain is no longer in a cortical level of thinking or using executive functioning...it is simply in protective mode. This may sound alarming, but it is somewhat like a wolf in the wild. The wolf reacts and responds on instinct and survival...you cannot rationalize with a wolf and ask it to sit for a treat or to choose the raw steak over your arm. Ok, ok...I am getting a little graphic here, but here's my point...this is the same type of reaction our sensory kiddos have. But unfortunately their little nervous systems often switch over to fight or flight, sometimes even daily. There has even been research done on this specific issue...the correlation between fight or flight and SPD.

### Why Do We See our Sensory Kids in "Fight or Flight"?

Children with sensory defensiveness or sensory over-registration perceive their environment as dangerous and painful based on how they process sensory information. Therefore their nervous system switches to the SNS and displays a "fight or flight" response.

### What Does "Fight or Flight" Look Like?

There are many different manifestations of "fight or flight" but some common responses may be:
- Kicking, screaming, biting, spitting, throwing things, etc.
- May try to find any place possible where visual and auditory input are decreased and where they will not be touched or required to make eye contact
- May try to find a tight space where the body will receive much needed proprioception and deep pressure touch (under a table or bed, buried in your arms, or retreating to the corner of a room)
- May cover their ears, close their eyes, and tuck their arms and legs in
- May run and try to escape from the situation at hand...without any regard to safety
- May lash out. (Keep in mind this is not the child being aggressive or hurtful, as the nervous system is doing the talking.)
- May scream, talk back, call names, cry uncontrollably (also the nervous system)
- May also present as "checking out" or zoning out
- Quick change in facial expression and quick shift of mood and emotion...possibly to irritability, frustration, anger, or crying and panic

## What Do You Do? How to Respond

- Encourage deep breathing...even if you are doing the deep breaths. It is amazing how the child will likely pick up on it and start taking deep breaths. Remember, talking to the child or asking the child to do it is not the ticket. The deep breaths will also help you as the parent feel better. Research indicates that taking deep breaths is one of the most effective tools to bring the brain/nervous system back to ready state.
- If the child will let you...just hold him/her tightly, providing deep pressure touch in the form of a uniform pressure bear hug. Do not rub the arm or back or hair. No rocking. Simply be quiet with them, taking deep breaths.
- Do not talk or try to rationalize or bargain with the child.
- If a sensory retreat is available, encourage or guide the child to go there.
- If the child has found a make-shift sensory retreat (behind a TV or under a bed), leave him/her alone until ready to come out. (It may take a while, be patient.)
- When the child is feeling better, follow up with a sensory activity involving proprioception (heavy/hard work) and resistive sucking/blowing/chewing...such as a bubble mountain or a chewy snack or smoothie. Continue to keep the environment quiet and calm for a while. If the child responds well to swinging, encourage calming rhythmical swinging.
- Keep taking deep breaths yourself :-)
- **As a proactive strategy, be sure you have sensory tools in place to address the types of sensory input which tend to trigger sensory overload, such as noise cancelling headphones or compression clothing to decrease input for tactile defensiveness.**

# Sensory Meltdowns

I think quite possibly the word **"meltdown"** is the most frequently used term and struggle for parents of sensory kiddos. A standard meltdown may be referring to a child who is kicking, screaming, biting, and/or spitting... or a child who simply can't stop crying....or a child reacting to a situation in a disruptive and aggressive manner... or a child seeking attention... or a child acting out to get his way....or a child who is simply losing all emotional control. Here's the thing. There is a difference between a STANDARD meltdown and a SENSORY meltdown.

**As a sensory OT I think the biggest missing puzzle piece is in understanding WHY a child has a meltdown.** Most parents, teachers, and caregivers simply have not been taught why the child has a meltdown and how to help. Unfortunately, meltdowns often fall into the behavior category in our society, which is the type I call standard meltdowns. Yet in my professional opinion, there is a very, very small percentage of meltdowns that warrant being considered behavioral, especially with our sensory kiddos! **IMPORTANT SENSORY CONCEPT: Children inherently want to please and do not want to misbehave or get in trouble.** I think this concept is SO very important to remember when talking about sensory meltdowns. The sensory meltdown is often misunderstood for attention seeking or spoiled behavior or simply the child trying to get what they want out of the situation. This may be true in a few cases, but with our sensory kiddos it is often much more deeply rooted than that. Here are some of the most common reasons a child may have a sensory meltdown....

- Sensory overload
- Dysregulation and the inability to maintain self-regulation and a ready state
- "Fight or flight" response to sensory overload, yet mistaken for a standard, behavior driven meltdown
- Inability to cope with a new or challenging situation
- Inability to communicate wants and needs
- Difficulty with transitions
- Lack of sleep or over tired
- Lack of proper nutrition or too much of the wrong food
- Change in routine

# Sensory or Behavior?

The question of "Is it sensory or behavior?" is the most common question I have been asked over the last 20 years as a sensory occupational therapist. Parents, teachers, and caregivers all have the same question, which is absolutely justified, as it can be a tough one. But what I have learned is to follow these steps....

### Scenario #1

FIRST look at the situation through "sensory goggles" vs. jumping to the conclusion that it is behavioral or attention seeking.

Next, analyze the situation at hand: Is the child displaying sensory signals such as covering ears or trying to escape from the current situation? Verbalizing that something is bothering him? Is it a chaotic situation? A new situation? A change in the normal routine?

If you answered yes to any of these questions, then remove the element which is possibly causing the child's response or reaction.

Offer the child a "sensory retreat" at that time.

If the above steps are taken and a positive change is <u>not</u> noted, then behavior may be considered.

### Scenario #2

A common so-called "behavior" is when a child is being fidgety . . . difficulty staying in a chair, touching others, and/or is easily distracted. These are the kids we call sensory seekers! They NEED to be moving and fidgeting with something to learn and need to be given a sensory tool or strategy to help them. This is crucial for their success in the classroom! This is definitely not a scenario of behavior...it is sensory! **<u>Very important:</u> These are usually the kids who have recess taken away from them as the consequence for their lack of attention or completion of a task...this is the exact opposite of what they need!** Recess will help feed their brain with the necessary sensory input needed in order to attend and learn.

### Scenario #3

Please consider the "fight or flight" response as a possibility when trying to determine sensory or behavior and refer to the previously discussed strategies.

# S.E.N.S.E. ©
## Making SENSE out of the situation!

Use this very simple strategy to help understand and address any challenging moment and when the question comes to your mind...is this sensory or behavior? How can I help my child?

- **S.** Stop, assess the situation, do not assume it is "behavior"
- **E.** Environment change
- **N.** Note the child's response to the environment change
- **S.** Sensory strategies and tools
- **E.** Embrace the positive and learn from the moment

### S.

**Stop.** Try not to simply react. It is important to analyze the situation to determine if there is a sensory trigger. Do not force the child through the situation, as this can create further negative reactions from the nervous system. Also, maintain a calm and objective state of mind, which will only benefit the situation. Sensory kiddos co-regulates via the people around them. If you are stressed or angry or panicked, this will create further dysregulation.

### E.

Change the **environment**, even if only briefly, as this can help you determine if there is indeed a sensory trigger. It will also give you another minute to assess the situation. And when I refer to changing the environment...this can simply be turning off the TV in the room, as the auditory input may be too much for the child.

### N.

**Notice** how the child responds to the change. Watch closely for body language, pattern of breathing, tone of voice, etc...this will tell you so much about the state of the nervous system. If you see a positive change, then you are on the right track; if not, change something else.

### S.

Implement **sensory strategies** right there on the spot. This could be deep pressure touch, a head compression, or letting your child bury his/her head into your chest while you give a bear hug. Or it could be offering a sensory retreat, a squish box, a weighted blanket or noise cancelling headphones. The sensory tool and strategy may be something as simple as a Camelbak® water bottle or encouraging deep breaths. It may also be leaving the group play date a little early, if needed. The list goes on and on....

### E.

**Embrace** the moment as a learning experience and develop a better understanding and respect for your child's sensory needs and differences. Do not let frustration get in the way by letting thoughts like "how do I fix this?" or writing it off as another bad experience. Learn from it...respond with respect....and embrace your child for who he/she is and will become. Remember that they simply want to be loved and understood.

# More Bang for Your Sensory Buck!

There are a few sensory integration techniques which I feel are often overlooked since they go back to "old school" sensory based therapy. I still believe they are crucial for sensory processing. In addition, applying these basic techniques can promote sensory processing even more effectively, as you will be working on multiple areas of development and sensory integration. Incorporating these four areas into treatment and into sensory home programs, as well as sensory activities at school, can have a significant impact on the brain for all children!

**Quality of Movement**
**Prone Extension**
**Full Body Flexion**
**Neck Extension**

## Quality of Movement

Assessing a child's quality of movement is a critical link in understanding sensory needs. The two biggest factors are prone extension and full body flexion, which will be addressed separately below. Quality of movement involves how the brain is "putting it all together" (sensory integration) and is shown through posture, upper body weight shifting and stability, shoulder stability, trunk control and core strength, lower body stability and weight shifting, trunk rotation, and body awareness.

- It is important as a therapist to assess these foundational skills prior to working on higher level function.
- It is important as a parent to be sure these areas are indeed assessed if the child is receiving occupational or physical therapy.
- It is important as a teacher to watch for signs of poor coordination, poor posture, or delays in gross/fine motor skills and refer to the school OT/PT for screening.

## Prone Extension

Prone extension is the "superman" position or the flying airplane position many of us did with our parents as children. The parent lies on the floor, lifting the child up in the air supporting the child at the belly while balancing and pretending to "fly like an airplane". Prone extension is very complex and often is taken for granted. The ability for the brain to coordinate the activation of ALL of the extensors in the body and then sustaining the movement is complex! Often when you ask a child with sensory processing dysfunction to assume this position, you will get a very uncoordinated display of extension. Asking the child to sustain that position can be nearly impossible. The most important thing to remember here is that it does not necessarily have to do with lack of strength! It is the lack of sensory integration and the ability to "put it all together".

Incorporating prone extension into sensory activities is an EXCELLENT way to promote sensory integration and sensory processing skills!

- Swinging in prone (on tummy)
- Scooter board in prone
- Going down a slide in prone
- Laying over a therapy ball and walking out with hands on the floor
- Jumping from a BOSU® ball and landing on belly on a soft landing pad
- Wheelbarrow walking

It is important to encourage arms and legs in full extension and reaching outward during these activities as well as lifting the head and looking forward! Make it fun and incorporate a catching, throwing, reaching game with these activities, as well.

**Full Body Flexion**
Full body flexion is the ability to lie on the floor on your back and then tuck your whole body into a ball. This includes tucking your chin and being able to hold your knees up close to your chin without holding them there with your hands. Your arms would be crossed on the chest in a relaxed fashion. This is just the opposite of prone extension. With full body flexion all of the flexor muscles of the body are activated. This is also very complex for the brain to "put it all together". The concepts of prone extension apply to full body flexion.

Incorporating full body flexion and extension into sensory activities is a POWERFUL way to promote sensory integration and sensory processing skills!
- Using swings such as a daisy disc swing or a bolster swing
- Lying backwards over a therapy ball and pulling up to a sitting position
- Sit-ups
- Jumping from a BOSU® ball tucked in a ball and landing on a soft landing pad
- Roly-Poly (tucking into a ball and rolling and rocking on the floor)
- Somersaults

**Neck Extension**
When the neck is in extension, the brain stem is activated. This facilitates the area in the brain that promotes self-regulation. Neck extension also helps develop visual motor skills. The neck is in extension when our body is in prone (on tummy) and we lift our head, which engages the muscles of the neck. If you think about it, the only time we spend a significant amount of time in prone with neck extension is as an infant during the developmental stages of rolling, propping on elbows, and then during crawling. It is important to continue these types of body positions through childhood to help the brain develop…and especially important for our sensory kiddos.

**Activity idea to promote neck extension…**
- Tummy time … propped up on elbows reading, working a puzzle, playing a board game, doing homework, etc.
- Crawling or bear crawling races
- Wheelbarrow walking
- Playing balloon volleyball on all fours
- Any of the prone extension activities mentioned above

# BONUS SECTION!

## The Survival Guide for Travelling with a Sensory Kiddo

For my precious sensory kiddos who were not able to find the joy and delight in a trip to the beach or an amusement park.

## Why is Travelling so Difficult?

Sensory kiddos love consistency, structure, and sameness. Their little world tends to be very scary, disorganized, and unpredictable…so routines and structure create a sense of comfort for the nervous system.

Actually, human beings in general like consistency, structure, and routine and often thrive in this type of environment. Think about the last time you slept in someone's guest room or in a hotel room. It was likely hard to fall asleep and get adjusted the first night. Or perhaps you woke up in the middle of the night, and it took a moment to come to your senses and remember where you were.

These types of challenges that we face when we travel are magnified and much more difficult for our sensory kiddos. Let's add to that the specific challenges that they face on a day to day basis even during their normal routine and environment . . . possibly hyper-sensitive to sounds and/or touch or craving constant movement or proprioception. Now imagine what even a weekend trip could do in regards to disruption of sensory processing.

Research suggests that it takes at least THREE TIMES as long for a sensory child to adjust to the new surroundings as it does the child with a neuro-typical brain. And not only that, when the child returns home, it will take THREE TIMES as long to get adjusted back to the normal daily routine!

I think we can all somewhat understand this as well, since I know for myself it is hard to get back into the normal daily routine after even a weekend trip. And it is much more difficult after a week or two of vacation.

Unfortunately, many places are not sensory friendly simply by nature. Even more unfortunate are the judgmental and uninformed people who give the disapproving looks when a child is melting down or just simply can't sit still on the airplane.

But we must move forward and educate and spread SPD awareness! And the best part is that our society is indeed starting to understand SPD and even the term "sensory" is being used more often and taken with acceptance and compassion rather than the "huh?" look on the person's face.

Through spreading awareness and understanding our sensory kiddos' needs in EVERY situation . . . including the hotel or the amusement park…we can improve their quality of life AND make for a pleasant trip or vacation for the whole darn family.

# Road Trip

**The oh-so-dreaded road trip....**
Hours of packing and preparing and loading the SUV with all of the snacks, coloring books, DVDs, and favorite pillows and blankies and it is time to hit the road! Only to encounter your first meltdown 30 minutes after jumping on the freeway. You tell yourself...why did we do this? I knew this would happen! This is going to be miserable (and a few other choice words). How will we possibly get through the next three days? Let's just turn around and go home.

But being the determined parent that you are, you keep on driving. Climbing over the front seat, bottom stuck to the roof of the car to try to reach the favorite stuffed animal that just got chucked during a moment of meltdown to then hopefully console and quiet the child. You sit back down in the passenger's seat and take a deep breath. "We can do this," you say in your head. Only to then hear the screech and scream of, "She hit me!". You turn back again and give a warning, "No hitting or we will turn around and go home!" You then offer more snacks or suggest a fun, keep-them-busy toy.

The screaming continues, the lashing out continues...and then comes the barf. (Sorry for the gross language, but it just seems so appropriate.) No warning, just a huge disgusting mess all over the clothes, the car seat, and the floor. Hopefully at least the sibling was spared.

You pull the SUV over to clean up the stinky mess, change the child's clothes, and console him. Everyone decides to get out for a stretch break and a potty break...then a few more deep breaths, and you hit the road again.

There are so many sensory factors and variables involved in a road trip. Of course every sensory kiddo has their unique sensory needs and differences, but I will discuss some of the most common sensory issues and then most importantly some suggestions on how to make the road trip a little more pleasant.

Let's start with...

**Strategic Positioning in the Vehicle**
Depending on the number of siblings involved, the age of the sensory kiddos, as well as the sensory needs and differences, the placement of the child can be crucial. Is the child sensitive to sound or touch? If so, and if possible, have the child positioned in the back and alone. If they are positioned right behind the front seats, then they get a whole lot of auditory input from siblings or others in the vehicle. Like sitting in the movie theater...if you are in the back you do not get all of the auditory distractions of those chomping popcorn or talking.

Although it may seem isolating to not have the child sit next to anyone, they will thank you in the long run. It will decrease the urge to touch or lash out at others, and on the opposite side of the coin, will decrease the chances of the child being touched or brushed against, which could cause a meltdown if tactile issues are present.

One last suggestion...if a parent can sit next to the child or an older sibling who understands the child's sensory needs and is a good sensory match . . . this would be a wise choice as well. Having a healthy sensory buddy next to you for deep pressure arm and hand rubs or being available to quietly interact with can be a wonderful thing.

### Tons of Sensory Breaks

I realize this may sound like a real hassle, but wouldn't it be better to be taking healthy sensory breaks rather than the REQUIRED negative road trip breaks?

I would suggest at least stopping once an hour…and not just for a potty break…I mean a real sensory break! Run, climb a tree, stop at a park, have wheelbarrow races at the rest area, move, move, move!

These ever-so-needed sensory breaks help everyone's brain regulate, but especially the sensory kiddo's brain. Movement breaks and added heavy/hard work (proprioception) breaks will help the child cope and maintain a ready state for continuation of the road trip.

### Oral Sensory Needs

Even if the child is not necessarily an oral seeker, meeting oral sensory needs while on a road trip are crucial for self-regulation. Of course, if the child is a sensory seeker, then be sure you have the oral sensory tools/chewies with you and definitely a backup or two! It is inevitable that on a trip the chewy gets lost! The best types of snacks for sensory kids are chewy or crunchy. Gum is great, as well, for children old enough to chew it. Stop for a milkshake or smoothie along the way too…the resistive sucking is excellent for self-regulation. A CamelBak® water bottle is my favorite for use with water in the car, as it has a great mouthpiece for chewing on and requires resistive sucking. Some kids like an oral sensory tool that vibrates, as it can be calming and soothing. You can even bring along a vibrating toothbrush!

### The Right Sensory Toys

Be sure you bring along your child's favorite fidget toys. More than one is best, with various textures and squeeze options…your child's sensory mood will change throughout the trip. Theraband® is an excellent tool to use in the car, and you can tie a piece to the door handle for your child to pull on for resistance and proprioception. Other great road trip sensory toys include Silly Putty®, Magna Doodle®, Lauri Toys Toddler Tote®, Lauri Toys Primer Pack®, Alex Toys My First Mosiac®, Melissa & Doug License Plate game®, and Wikki Stix®.

### Sensory Tools

Depending on your child, there will be a few essential sensory tools that will make for a much more enjoyable trip. These tools may include earplugs, noise cancelling headphones, an MP3 player with the child's favorite soothing music, a weighted lap pad or blanket, a compression vest, sunglasses, wide brimmed hat, vibrating pillow, and of course the oral sensory tools already mentioned.

### Meals

I know it is so tempting to just whip through the drive-thru and get the adored chicken nuggets…but if possible, only do this in moderation on the trip. Pack as much food as you can with healthier options full of protein and not full of preservatives, additives, and dyes. Pack crunchy carrot sticks and apples as an alternative, or turkey jerky is awesome, too. Often the food your child eats on a trip can be the culprit to the sensory dysregulation and meltdowns. The best sensory option is the drive-thru where you can get a smoothie or a milkshake!

**Bathroom Breaks and Bathroom Urgency**
Sensory kiddos often have a difficult time registering the need to go to the bathroom until the very last minute. This is due to the interoceptors in the gut (like proprioceptors) having a difficult time giving sensory feedback to the brain in regards to "it's time to go potty". It is important to respect this with sensory children, and know that if they suddenly say….I GOTTA GO POTTY! …they mean it. During those ever so frequent sensory breaks you are going to take, use those also as an opportunity to go to the bathroom. But please be tolerant and understanding if your trip requires yet another potty stop.

**The Dreaded…I am gonna throw up.**
I saved the best for last. Car sickness is very much linked to sensory processing difficulties, especially if the child has difficulty with processing vestibular input (movement). Being in a car becomes extra difficult for a sensory kiddo when there a lot of starts and stops, as well as a curvy road. Usually a sensory child is not able to read or attend visually to something due to this vestibular issue. A few tips that may help include:
- Cover the window the child is sitting next to with a pillow case. This decreases the peripheral visual input which can trigger car sickness.
- Position the child in the car so he can see directly out the front window (middle seat).
- Avoid riding sideways or backwards, which are sometimes present in trucks and SUVs.
- Providing an oral sensory tool or Camelbak® water bottle to suck on with water or a sour beverage.
- Lemon drops are known to help nausea.
- Travel at night when the child is sleeping, so the eyes are closed and the visual component is not a trigger.
- Using other sensory tools which the child typically responds well to can also be helpful.
- Don't forget the barf bag or bucket….sensory kiddos often are unable to give you warning when it is time to throw up.

# Airplanes

I must first begin by saying I wish there were more understanding, empathetic, and compassionate people in this world. It is one thing to have a not so nice person living down the street, or passing someone in the grocery store who gives you a glare when your child is having a sensory meltdown…but an AIRPLANE?! Could there be a worse place for Mrs. Grumpy Pants?!

The close quarters and "tight spaces" may be wonderful for sensory kiddos at home…but the airplane is the last "tight space" a sensory child wants to be in. There are soooooooooooo many factors which make air travel difficult.

- Lack of vestibular and proprioceptive input, and the inability to get it when they need it
- Unfamiliar and unpredictable auditory input, such as airplane bathroom toilet flushing sound
- Unpleasant sensations such as ears popping, and possible internal discomfort when the plane is taking off and landing due to vestibular intolerance
- LONG periods of time required to be seated
- So many restrictions and rules to follow
- Parents a little stressed and not in the most relaxed state of mind to help the sensory kiddo (possibly because of the Mrs. Grumpy Pants on board)
- Uncomfortable airplane seats, not conducive to the soft, nest-like feel that a sensory child needs
- Limited options for play and activities
- Did I mention Mrs. Grumpy Pants?

**Let's Make the Most Out of It**
Since air travel is sometimes just necessary, all we can do is cope, adapt, tolerate, and be prepared with sensory tools and strategies!

Many of the recommendations I made in the ROAD TRIP chapter also apply on the airplane…but I will list them here again for ease of reading.

**In the Airport**
If your child is a sensory seeker, now is the time to let him/her run, hop, skip, jump, etc! This is needed to help self-regulate when on the plane. Please do not discourage it! Also, bring along a stroller even for a little bit older kids…a jogging stroller is ideal, for a portable sensory retreat. A jogging stroller is the best because it wraps around the child's body and provides deep pressure touch. It also typically has a canopy over it, over which you can then drape a blanket to create a cozy tent feeling in the stroller. This is your portable sensory retreat. You can then add a weighted blanket, weighted lap pad, oral sensory tools, fidget toy, and other appropriate sensory tools. Believe me, you will not only be using this portable sensory retreat in the airport, but it will also come in handy along the trip many times.

**Strategic Positioning on the Airplane**
Depending on the number of siblings involved and the age of the sensory kiddos as well as their sensory needs and differences, the placement of the sensory child is crucial. Is the child sensitive to touch? If so, and if possible, have the child positioned at the window seat. Sitting in the center or on the aisle is much more difficult for those not liking to be touched or brushed against. Be sure the

most appropriate family member is sitting next to the sensory child, even if requested otherwise! If a parent can sit next to the child or an older sibling…one who understands the child's sensory needs and is a good sensory match . . . this would be best. Having a healthy sensory buddy next to you for deep pressure arm and hand rubs or being available to quietly interact with can be a wonderful thing.

If possible, request at check in or when you make the reservation to be seated in the front. (I know this is opposite of what I suggested for a road trip, but I will explain). The closer you are to the front…the very front seats would be ideal…the less effect the possible crying/screaming/loud sounds your child may make will have on others. This is very stressful for parents and such a big worry on the plane. You can request this at check in and be sure to mention that you have a child with special needs and accommodations due to sensory processing disorder. The airline staff will likely do their best to accommodate. Don't be afraid to explain the scenario a little bit to them and let them know how making the accommodations can help everyone!

**Creating a Sensory Break**
As we know, this is extremely limited, but here are a few suggestions that can help:

- Prior to boarding the plane, make sure that the sensory kiddo gets a powerful dose of vestibular and proprioceptive input…5-10 minutes will do. Let the child run in the airport or march, hop, jump, etc. If there are stairs around, encourage climbing them a few times. Hang your child upside down for a minute. (Inverting the head is excellent vestibular input!) Wheelbarrow walk the child around a little. Who cares if people look at you weird! You are advocating and doing what is best for your child's sensory needs!
- Also be sure to make time for a sensory break during a layover during the trip! Refrain from asking your child to sit and wait at the gate…let them move, move move! Yes, it takes some effort to supervise, but you will thank me later.
- When it is safe to do so during flight, let your child pace the aisle for a little while…it can at least get the wiggles out a tiny bit. And once again, don't worry about what Mrs. Grumpy Pants is thinking.
- While in the seat (and it is safe to unbuckle) have your child squat in the seat, do chair push-ups, even let them stand for a minute if they are small enough. I would even recommend letting them do a headstand in the seat (it really would be good for them!), but I bet this would send the flight attendant through the roof of the plane.

**Oral Sensory Needs**
Even if the child is not necessarily an oral seeker, meeting oral sensory needs while on the airplane is crucial for self-regulation. Of course, if the child is a sensory seeker, then be sure you have his/her oral sensory tool/chewy with you and definitely a backup or two! It is inevitable that on a trip the chewy gets lost! The best types of snacks for sensory kids are chewy or crunchy. Gum is great as well for children old enough to chew it…and is also excellent for helping those painful popping ears. Purchase a milkshake or smoothie prior to boarding or during a layover…the resistive sucking is excellent for self-regulation. A CamelBak® water bottle is my favorite for use with water on the plane as it has a great mouthpiece for chewing on and it requires resistive sucking. Just watch out! The pressure in the plane can make the water squirt out a little…and possibly alarming for your little one. Some kids like an oral sensory tool that vibrates, and it can be calming and soothing. You can even bring along a vibrating toothbrush!

### The Right Sensory Toys
Be sure to bring along your child's favorite fidget toys (more than one is best) with various textures and squeeze options…your child's sensory mood will change throughout the trip. Theraband® is an excellent tool to use on the airplane, and you can tie a piece to the arm rest and your child can pull on it for the resistance and proprioception. Other great airplane sensory toys include Silly Putty®, Magna Doodle®, Lauri Toys Toddler Tote®, Lauri Toys Primer Pack®, Alex Toys My First Mosiac®, and Wikki Stix®. A portable DVD player is not a bad idea at all in this scenario either, especially if your child "gets in the zone" with a favorite movie.

### Sensory Tools
Depending on your child, there will be a few essential sensory tools that will make for a much more tolerable plane ride. These tools may include earplugs or noise cancelling headphones, an MP3 player with the child's favorite soothing music, a weighted lap pad or blanket, a compression vest, sunglasses, wide brimmed hat, vibrating pillow, and of course the oral sensory tools already mentioned. The auditory tools may also be needed for sensory kiddos who typically wouldn't need them…there is such a large amount of unpredictable auditory input on an airplane. The sunglasses and hat may be necessary to help create somewhat of a "faux sensory retreat" due to all of the social demands involved with being on a plane. Let the child cope a little better with all of the sensations and the strange surroundings by staying under the big hat and sunglasses…its ok…it's not the time to work on social skills…I promise you that one.

### The Special Gadgets on the Airplane
The airplane is full of fun little buttons and levers that you only see on an airplane. It's OKAY if your child wants to open and close and open and close the window shade and the tray! It really is. Please refrain from choosing this battle. The person in front of you would have a lot more to contend with if you insist on not touching the fun little levers and such.

The buttons above you…go ahead and let your child explore them once instead of saying they are off limits…let him get it out of the system. Keep in mind the air knob may cause a reaction for some kiddos if they struggle with tactile defensiveness, and the air blowing on their little face may be painful. Please also keep this in mind when they are seated…the air may be a sensory trigger for problems.

In the bathroom…all sorts of fun things to explore in there! Again…let them explore the faucet and the paper towels and tissues…not the toilet though! Back away from the toilet! (If indeed that were really possible in there.) But seriously, this may sound horrible and wrong…but after your child goes to the bathroom, do NOT flush it. Return to your seat, and if you feel so inclined to go back and flush it without your child, then go for it. Even with your child standing right outside the door, it can be so loud that the flushing could trigger sensory overload.

### The Dreaded Airplane Meltdown
Just be prepared and expect at least one meltdown or at least a little sensory dysregulation out of your child. It will likely happen, so if you are prepared and expecting it…it can go a little smoother. Hopefully with the advice and suggestions I have given, your sensory kiddo will have the sensory tools and strategies to help get through the trip. But there is always the unexpected "bumps in the

road/air" (literally) that are unpredictable and simply out of our control. If this does happen here are my suggestions:

- Remain calm. Your child will feed off of your stress and response to the situation. Be the solid and regulated rock that they need at that moment.
- Provide deep pressure touch or a bear hug and sit quietly with the child. Do not try to quiet her with words or rationalize with her...it will only make the situation worse and last longer.
- Offer an oral sensory tool…this is a very good way to help soothe and calm the child.
- If there is a sensory trigger that can be removed or addressed at the moment, assess the situation and respond accordingly.
- Create a makeshift sensory retreat using a blanket or weighted blanket if you brought one…cover the child entirely with the blanket and provide gentle pressure to the body. Hopefully they will have tried to curl up in flexion (like fetal position). Flexion is the most organizing type of input.
- Use noise cancelling headphones if you have them.

**Not the Time to Work on Social Graces**

Please try to refrain from showing the world that you are a great parent and that you have taught your child manners. This is not the time for your child to initiate or engage in a conversation with the flight attendant or the guy at security, nor is it the time to request even a simple please or thank you. Just let your child be quiet, bury his head in your chest, or hide under a blanket or hat to avoid eye contact. It's ok, it really is. All that really matters during this time is that your sensory kiddo stays as regulated as possible and avoids sensory overload. Insisting on manners and social interaction can create dysregulation and sensory overload in a time like this.

# Staying with Relatives or Friends

Most of us personally have a story or have heard a story about the uncle, mother-in-law, or a friend who thinks they have all of the answers to parenting. Now bring in the sensory factor and you just created your worst nightmare.

Educating those around us about SPD and sensory differences is the very best strategy in advocating for our sensory kiddos. And this is an absolutely crucial link when you are visiting and/or staying with friends or relatives.

My first suggestion is prior to the visit, begin your SPD awareness campaign with your hosts! You choose the best avenue based on the individual...it may be a phone call and discussion about SPD and the possible situations that may arise during the visit. It may be mailing a sensory handbook to them, such as *Understanding Your Child's Sensory Signals*, which is easy to read and makes sense to those not so familiar with SPD. If you send them something too wordy and complicated, it won't get read . . . simple as that. Perhaps an email or letter explaining the upcoming visits and some of the modifications that may need to be made would be effective.

Now if you do not feel the friends or relatives are going to be receptive to this, then stay somewhere else. It is going to be difficult for your sensory kiddo staying away from home as it is, and you do NOT need the added stress of someone possibly not respecting your child's sensory differences and needs.

**Assess Your Surroundings**
Upon arrival to your new temporary landing pad, it will be important to determine if there are any specific sensory triggers which may be a challenge . . . such as a jumping, barking dog. Adapt as needed. Encourage the use of noise cancelling headphones and talk with your kiddo about a possible plan to limit the unexpected jumps from the dog.

Look for your prime sensory tools as well...maybe a trampoline in the backyard or a therapy ball in the house. You will want to show your child where the appropriate places will be to get crucial sensory input. If it is not really a kid-friendly house, then it will be necessary to come up with a game plan with the host. Based on your child's sensory needs, discuss this with the host and come up with a plan.

**Sleeping Arrangements**
This is probably the most challenging part for sensory kiddos, yet the most important to address. If your child uses a weighted blanket, be sure to bring it along on the trip. If you use music or white noise, bring this as well. Since staying in an unfamiliar house is difficult for all of us, be sure to make a special cozy little sensory retreat for your child to sleep in. (The retreat will be multi-purpose.) Create a cozy corner with lots of pillows and blankets or make a squish box with supplies in the home. If you are lucky enough that your host has a twin size duvet cover, make a pillow cave as well!

For the pillow cave: using the twin size duvet...fill it up with blankets, pillows, and stuffed animals...let the child go inside as a sensory retreat. At bedtime, fluff it up in the corner of a room and have your child sleep on it like a nest. Of course this is only recommended for children who are mobile and able to maneuver their body safely in the nest.

For the squish box: use a large plastic tote or laundry basket….just the right size container for your child to sit in and get squished a little. Add a couple blankets and pillows to make it cozy. This provides full body deep pressure touch and proprioception to help the child's nervous system regulate.

Another option for a weighted blanket is to use a heavy quilt or denim blanket folded into a large square, just the right size to drape over your child. Folding it creates a dense, heavy blanket.

Make sure you have brought along your child's favorite blanket, oral sensory tool, cuddle toy, and any other important sensory tool that helps her sleep.

And last, but not least, be sure to provide full body deep pressure touch/squeezes at bedtime. This will help your child's nervous system transition to sleep easier in an unfamiliar place.

### Mealtime

Sensory kiddos often struggle with food issues already…and then you add the "have to sit still" factor and the social interaction with those at the table. This is likely going to be much more challenging during your visit. The child may not be comfortable with the people at the table, it may be louder than usual. The food may be different than what is typically served at home. All of these components can create a real sensory challenge for your child! Please be sensitive to this and respectful of the fact that it may be incredibly difficult to face all of these different components of mealtime.

Here are my suggestions…

- Prior to the group situation, prepare the child's nervous system with a 15-minute movement and heavy/hard work activity.
- Keep in mind that 10-15 minutes at the dinner table will likely be the maximum amount of time the child can handle. A kid friendly side table with a ball chair as the seat would be best, or just the kid friendly table.
- Asking the child to try new foods during an already challenging sensory experience may be out of the question. The child's nervous system is already stressed. Provide safe and comforting healthy foods that the child likes. I know, you may get some "feedback" on this one…this is one of the topics you can discuss prior to the visit.

### Socializing and Playtime

Socializing and interacting with unfamiliar adults and playing with unfamiliar children will indeed be a huge challenge for your sensory kiddo. There can be so many factors and variables…

- The pitch, frequency, speed of speech, and volume of sound of those around the child may be overwhelming to the child. Be sure to be sensitive to this and modify as needed. The child may need more frequent sensory retreat breaks or possibly earplugs or noise cancelling headphones. Keep in mind this may be a

factor during the trip, even though auditory input may not typically affect the child.
- The amount of touch and type of touch given by those around them is also a factor. Constant hugs, love pats, or kisses may be just too much for them. These are usually coming in at a greater rate than on a typical day.
- The type of interaction during play may be a challenge. Is the other child "in your face" or very active and overwhelming in play? Does he like to constantly wrestle or play too rough?
- On the other hand…maybe your child is the one being the "in your face and space" and constantly wanting to wrestle. Make sure the other child involved is a good match for this.
- Do not insist on eye contact, hugs/kisses, or even verbal communication while your child is being introduced or interacting with new and unfamiliar people. This is incredibly difficult for sensory kiddos. More information on this topic is found in *Understanding Your Child's Sensory Signals*.

**A Sensory Retreat**
A sensory retreat will be a crucial component during your stay with relatives or friends. Your sensory child may need this retreat on a regular basis during your stay and should indeed be the safe place to retreat to during sensory overload, fight or flight, or just when needing a place to re-group, re-set, and get a nice dose of proprioception.

You can create a sensory retreat with household items. Be creative! You can also use the jogging stroller which was discussed in the AIRPLANE chapter for those children small enough to use it. Here are a few other ideas…
- A squish box in a nice quiet and dim room. Make the squish box with a laundry basket or plastic tote, add blankets and pillows and have your child "squish into it". Add a favorite fidget toy, an oral sensory tool, or a weighted item as well.
- A pillow cave, which you may be using for sleep as well. You may need to bring the twin size duvet cover from home…but then add pillows and blankets and soft items from the host's home. Have the child go inside the pillow cave, or fluff it up in the corner of a room and have the child get cozy on it like a nest. Add the same items as listed for the squish box.
- Drape a blanket over a small table and place this in a quiet room. Add cozy and comfortable items underneath the table, including other sensory tools.
- A cozy quiet spot in a walk-in closet can work, as well.

**Keeping Somewhat of a Routine**
I realize this is easier said than done. But please, please, please try your best to keep somewhat of a routine! Our sensory kiddos THRIVE on it! And it can make all of the difference in self-regulation and the child's ability to cope with all of the new sensory input and new environment during the stay!

**Sensory Tools**
I have already mentioned quite a few sensory tools to be utilized during your stay with relatives or friends. And since you have likely travelled to this location via plane or car…then you already have your sensory tools with you! Whooo hoooo!

# Hotels

### What to Look for in a Hotel
Here are a few starting suggestions when you are choosing your hotel. Even though it may cost a little more, it will likely make your stay a whole lot more pleasant. And nothing is more helpful than a good night's sleep for your sensory kiddo and the rest of the family.

- Stay away from rooms with a wall unit for heat and air conditioning. I know these are very common, but many hotels have a central heating and air conditioning system. This can be so helpful since the constant auditory input of it turning on/off can keep a sensory child up all night.
- Be sure the hotel has a pool...this may indeed be your sensory saving grace during the hotel stay.
- Some outdoor space for running around would be ideal. Or at least a kid friendly hotel where the child can run up and down the halls a little.

### Check-In Requests
It is important to be pro-active and prepare as much as possible for staying at a hotel. This preparation begins when you book your room reservation. If you wait until check-in for special requests, the hotel may not be able to honor them based on availability, so be sure to address them when you book your room! Here are my suggestions for special requests....

- Request a quiet room away from the elevator, any freeway noise, or any common areas. Sensory kiddos often hear everything.
- Request a rollaway bed and a bunch of extra pillows and even an extra comforter (not just the cheap flimsy blankets) that you can push up into the corner of the room and create a cozy nest for some extra proprioception. Do not be afraid to ask for as many as you think your child may need!
- If your child is small enough, bring along a pack and play and create a nice cozy nest in there for your child to sleep in.

### Sleeping Arrangements
Based on those suggestions, create the most conducive place for your sensory child to sleep. Sleeping with a sibling might not be the best idea. Paying a little extra money for the rollaway bed will very likely be worth it. Also be sure to bring along a weighted blanket if you have one, your child's most comfortable jammies, and also a white noise machine or a music player with the normal bedtime music. The key is to keep as many things as consistent with home as possible. Sensory kiddos thrive on consistency and routine! It will be well worth it to haul along the extra items and take the extra steps. The alternative may be a grumpy and dysregulated child.
**Try very hard to stay on the normal home sleep schedule during your entire trip.**

### The Pool
Swimming is an excellent tool for much needed proprioception. Proprioceptive input is regulating, organizing, and calming. You will most likely want to use the pool as a sensory tool during your stay. Choose quiet times at the pool so the sensory tool doesn't backfire on you. Often right when the pool opens in the morning around 10am is a great time, and this is also an effective way to prep your child's nervous system for the day. Don't forget to bring the goggles from home!

### Sensory Breaks
Now I know if any hotel owners or companies get hold of this book, they will go through the roof…but a little bit of supervised jumping on the beds is excellent for the nervous system.

Hopefully the hotel has an outdoor play area, but if not, then maybe some wheelbarrow or crab walking in the hallway and some running up and down the stairs will do the brain some good. You have to get creative with your sensory breaks and activities in the hotel. Sometimes the workout rooms have large exercise balls…if so, you can request to borrow one to use with your child. If you explain your situation, the hotel staff will likely be accommodating.

## The Beach

The beach can be a wonderful, peaceful, memorable experience of a lifetime for a child…but this can be a whole different story for a sensory kiddo. It may seem very peaceful and relaxing, but there are SO many sensory factors that come into play. As a parent, it is important to see this experience through your "sensory goggles" and determine which sensory triggers may be an issue for your child.

### The Sand

Now if you have a sensory seeker at heart who loves tactile experiences, than you have it made! Your little sensory seeker is going to dig, bury, roll, run, and jump in the sand. And it can also be an excellent proprioceptive and heavy/hard work activity while playing in the sand, which will help regulate and calm the nervous system. On the other hand…sometimes a child who typically enjoys different textures may indeed have difficulty with the sand because of the overwhelming amount of sensory input involved and the amount of sand on the beach. The beach is quite different than just a sandbox. So it is important to be prepared for whatever sensory twist may come your way. Here are some helpful tips….

- Do NOT just plop your child down into the sand in bare feet and a swimming suit or swimming trunks! Begin by sitting the child in a low to the ground beach chair, and let the child lead the way. If and when they are ready to explore the texture, they will. Do NOT force it.
- If your child is extremely tactilely defensive, I would recommend nice snug neoprene water shoes which cover the feet and give deep pressure.
- Provide plenty of sand tools so the child can first explore the sand that way.
- Wet sand and dry sand have completely different textures…offer the opportunity for both. Your child may tolerate one better than the other.
- I would also suggest a rash guard shirt for girls and boys to cover their chest/trunk if they are defensive to the sand. Rash guards also serve as a compression garment which will provide regulating proprioception during your time at the beach. A snug fitting life jacket is not only a great tool for safety, but it also provides deep pressure/compression as well!
- Having your child wear goggles while playing in the sand is not a bad idea either, since even a tiny bit of sand near or in the eye can send a sensory kiddo into fight or flight.

### The Wind

Wind is often a factor at the beach…especially on the Pacific Ocean in the northwest! Wind can be especially noxious and uncomfortable for sensory children…because it is unpredictable, comes in different strengths, and in this case, can blow the sand. OUCH! One little grain of sand blown at a sensory kiddo's face can be extremely painful and scary. Here are my suggestions…

- Avoid the beach on a super windy day…it just simply isn't worth it. Breezy is ok, but real windy will likely be just way too much if your child is a sensory avoider.
- The sensory tools I recommend are a rash guard and a sweatshirt or wind breaker with a hood, if it is one of the cooler days. Earplugs or noise cancelling headphones can be helpful, as well as sunglasses or goggles and a big floppy hat with a chin strap, of course.

### The Sun
The sun can be very draining for all of us at the beach, and you guessed it, even more draining for a sensory kiddo. The sun may also be way too bright for your child, so it is important to be prepared for this. Here are some ideas to help...

- Polarized sunglasses
- Big floppy hat
- Portable umbrella for shade
- Sun screen, of course
- Rash guard
- Tons of drinking water...not sweetened drinks or juice, and definitely not soda pop

### The Water
The ocean is obviously quite different than the pool. So keep in mind your little sensory swimmer may not be as fond of the ocean. All it takes is for one little thing to be different...and the idea of swimming is out of the question for a sensory kiddo. The ocean is in constant motion with waves in all different sizes, and the water looks different, smells different, and tastes different. There are two scenarios which I want to bring up....

If you have an extreme sensory seeker you MUST be so cautious and careful with a watchful eye. A sensory seeker can get in a "sensory tunnel" and if the ocean looks just way too inviting, then all safety and judgment blows away in the breeze. Even if you call for the child to stop or come back, he may truly may not process it and "hear" you.

On the other hand, a sensory avoider may be downright scared and overwhelmed. Do not force the issue...it will be a huge accomplishment for the child to simply put his feet in the water and experience the waves. If the child does want to wade a little more and lay in the wet sand near the edge of the waves, goggles and swimmers earplugs are strongly recommended.

### Best Beach Activities for a Sensory Kiddo
After now completing this section, you see that the beach can be a challenging place for a sensory child. But it can be a successful and pleasant experience with the right sensory knowledge and tools.

Every sensory kiddo is different and it will take wearing your "sensory goggles" to determine which sensory experiences the child is avoiding and seeking out at the beach. But involving proprioception is a great idea no matter what. So running on the beach, digging in the sand, walking through the deep sand, and frolicking in the waves and doing a little swimming are all excellent proprioceptive activities.

### A Portable Sensory Retreat
For a child who is small enough...probably through the toddler ages...you can bring along a Pack N Play® type playpen to set up on the beach and fill it with some soft pillows and a blanket, and then cover the whole thing with a lightweight sheet. This can serve as a nice sensory retreat. If you brought the jogging stroller on the trip, it can also be a good portable retreat as previously discussed.

# Camping and Hiking

### The Campsite
Camping provides so many wonderful opportunities for sensory exploration, especially tactile input. For the sensory seekers, it will be important to determine exploration boundaries, and even then a close watchful eye will be needed since the child may get in that "sensory tunnel" and keep on exploring. For the sensory avoiders…bring along some child-size gardening gloves so they can enjoy exploring as well. Also bringing along a bucket for gathering "treasures" provides a heavy work activity, and it also decreases frustration for children who try to gather in their little hands every stick, pinecone, and stone they find. Sensory kiddos tend to be real gatherers of treasures.

The campfire will be very tempting for the sensory seeker. So my suggestion is to incorporate a heavy/hard work activity to help create a safe boundary for them. Usually a fire pit has some sort of boundary, but I suggest creating a ring around the perimeter of the fire pit with appropriately large rocks, at a greater distance than normal. Your child will love helping with this fun and regulating task!

### Tools for Sleeping
Sleeping in a tent or camper is difficult for many of us, and will likely be extra difficult for your sensory child. Earplugs or noise cancelling headphones is the first thing that comes to my mind. The night time sounds are one of the most unique sensory components of camping….and often sensory kiddos hear EVERYTHING. As discussed in previous sections…you will want to bring along as many of your child's normal sensory tools for sleep. And if sleeping in a tent, be extra diligent in providing a soft, cozy surface for your child to sleep on. The sleeping bag will also likely be your child's best friend and may even be a little sensory retreat during the camping trip.

### Explore, Explore, Explore
Take this opportunity to let your sensory seeker go for it! What a beautiful time and place to let your child dig in the dirt, touch all of the different textures of plants and trees, discover new little bugs and critters, run/climb/skip/hop and simply explore their sensory world! Try your very best to be mindful of this and put as few restrictions in place as possible…of course, safety and respect for nature comes first, but then let them EXPLORE!!!!

### Hiking
Hiking is an absolutely awesome activity for self-regulation! Hiking involves a HUGE amount of proprioception. Encourage your child to climb hills and rocks and jump off of rocks and logs. This is great for body awareness, balance, and overall gross motor development. Also, encourage your child to walk on logs!

I would suggest hiking at times during your camping trip when you feel your child may need a dose of self-regulating and calming input. Yet I would caution you . . . it is important to gauge and monitor the distance of the hike…or you may be "backpacking" your kiddo back to the campsite. It is very common for a sensory kiddo to be "hot or cold"…when they are done, they are done. Period.

Speaking of backpacks…for the little ones, hiking can still be a wonderful sensory experience while being carried in the infant/toddler packs. The child will experience a great amount of full body deep pressure touch and also vestibular input during the hike. But be sure to let the little one out for moments of hiking and sensory exploration, as well.

It is very important to bring plenty of water while hiking, and my favorite tool in this case is the Camelbak® water bottle, which comes in all sizes! There are also Camelbak® water backpacks which have an excellent mouthpiece for an oral sensory tool and the backpack comes in adult and child sizes.

## Amusement Parks

Let me first begin by mentioning that if it is at all possible, schedule your trip to an amusement park on the OFF SEASON. This can make such a difference in the overall experience.

**The Classic Multi-Sensory Environment**
Multi-sensory experiences, even the grocery store, can be overwhelming and very difficult for a sensory kiddo. Now an amusement park takes it to a whole new level.

Let's begin with visual input….so much to take in from all of the colorful rides and displays, possibly large dressed up characters, and all of the people walking around. So much to see and take in from the visual side of things…AND the sunlight, as well.

Next would be auditory input…this can be a REAL challenge. Music, unexpected and unpredictable buzzing and beeping sounds, children screaming and squealing in delight, people talking, loud announcements on the rides, etc.

Tactile input…this can simply be difficult from walking from one ride to the next. People brushing and bumping against you, constantly in your "personal bubble".

Vestibular input…lots of walking and possibly riding in a stroller or wagon or in a backpack just scratches the surface of all of the possible movement experiences which may be in store throughout the day. Where else are you going to experience movement in all possible body positions and in every plane and direction of movement, at all different speeds?

**The Rides**
It is important to remember that each and every ride is not just the actual ride itself. It is also a combination of sensory input typically involving all of the senses mentioned above, along with the component of the unknown, unpredictability, anticipation, and the possibility of sensory overload and the inability to tolerate the new vestibular experience.

If your child is a sensory seeker, then this may be a little easier, except for the fact that even a sensory seeker can develop sensory overload in a new multi-sensory experience like this. Vestibular input is extremely powerful and this must be respected and taken into consideration for all children at an amusement park. Watch for signs of sensory overload including systemic reactions such as flushing of the face, nausea, fever, etc.

For a sensory avoider or a child who has difficulty with tolerating movement, an amusement park is NOT the place to work on tolerating movement. Be prepared for this, and trying to talk the child into it or bribing her is actually very unfair to your sensory kiddo. Simply respect the fact that if she says no, she means no.

For all sensory children, spending time on the calming rides can be very beneficial, such as the monorail or train. This can provide a necessary dose of calming and regulating input and help the brain sort out all of the intense sensory input the child has been trying to process.

Also, be sure to utilize the play areas where your child can get a good dose of proprioception from climbing, hanging, jumping, etc. Many of the big theme parks have huge climbing structures and play zones for children.

### Standing in Line

We all know standing in line at an amusement park is not an easy task for any of us! Just imagine how it may feel for a little sensory seeker. Hanging on the bars while waiting in line really is ok…matter of fact it is good for them. Hanging provides joint traction to the arms (proprioception), which is regulating, calming, and organizing. This is also a great time to hold your child and let him play some monkey games by hanging from your arms or hanging upside down while you hold the feet. Also try the panda bear game with your child latched onto your leg and see how long they can hang on. Change his perspective…have the child sit on your shoulders or give him a piggy back ride! This is also a good time to pull out some of your sensory tools in your travel bag…such as a fidget toy, music with headphones, oral sensory tool, and the Camelbak® water bottle, or even a crunchy or chewy snack.

Now for the sensory avoider, standing in line is downright difficult. The close proximity of the people brushing against the child by accident, in addition to the auditory and visual input, can be overwhelming. Do not be surprised if your child wants to simply be held and bury her face against your body. This is a good time to use noise cancelling headphones or an MP3 player with soft calming music. A big floppy hat and sunglasses may also be helpful if the child is overwhelmed by all of the visual input and potential eye contact from others.

The good part about all of this is that many amusement/theme parks now offer a fast track pass or guest assistance card or other options and modifications for those with special needs. This includes SPD, of course. But often there is even a long wait in the alternate line…so it may be helpful to use some of the ideas listed above.

Another thing to keep in mind and respect for your child is that he may wait in line and say he wants to go on the ride, but it may be a whole different story when it is your turn. You may need to stand there and let others in front of you, over and over again, as the transition from standing in line to the anticipation of getting on a ride with unknown and unpredictable sensory input may be completely overwhelming. Try to be patient. Take deep breaths…both of you. And even let the rest of the family go ahead while one parent or adult waits with the child until ready. Keep in mind that your child might not get to the point of being ready, and you may need to walk away. Respect this and accept it…if you get frustrated, this will only lead to further difficulty with self-regulation for your sensory kiddo.

### Social Interaction

Do not ask your child to make eye contact or talk to the staff or others nearby. This is an extremely difficult time for your kiddo and is not the time to work on social interaction.

### A Portable Sensory Retreat

The good ol' jogging stroller, wagon, or other type of stroller which I talked about in previous sections will likely be your best friend on your amusement park adventure. It will be your sensory kiddo's safe place and mini/portable sensory retreat. The main components of the portable sensory retreat need to be:

- Cozy and squishy (lots of blankets and a stuffed animal or pillow)
- A blanket to cover the entire stroller to minimize all sensory input
- Something weighted if possible, such as a weighted lap pad or blanket
- Fidget toy and possibly a vibrating toy or vibrating pillow
- Oral sensory tools
- Crunchy and chewy snacks
- Earplugs or noise cancelling headphones, MP3 player with soft and calming music, possibly a floppy hat and sunglasses

You will want to use this sensory retreat often and throughout the day…not just when your child is in sensory overload. Be pro-active about it and use it as a place to re-group and help your sensory kiddo self-regulate. Use it between rides, anytime you are doing a lot of waiting, and any time your child seems to need it or request it!

**Sensory Tools**
Once again…you have likely travelled by car or by plane and already have your sensory tools! Just be sure you bring them along to the amusement park. It may seem like extra work and a hassle, but you will be so happy you hauled it all with you. Here is a list of the essentials….

- Portable sensory retreat
- Oral sensory tools and Camelbak® water bottle
- Earplugs or noise cancelling headphones
- Floppy hat and/or sunglasses
- Compression clothing
- And lots and lots of bear hugs and deep pressure touch all day long

**Food and Drink**
If your child is sensitive to food dyes, additives and preservatives, or is on a GF/CF diet, then a restricted diet is required. The park will need to allow for you to bring in special foods for the restricted diet.

If your child is not on a restricted diet, please note that most, if not all, sensory kiddos are very sensitive to food dyes, preservatives, sugars, and are usually carb cravers. Even though the amusement park is often the time that children are given all sorts of treats, it is important to balance this and keep it limited. Focus on the protein rich foods and bring along snacks that are crunchy or chewy such as apples, carrot sticks, cheese sticks, fruit leather, etc. And try to stick to water as the drink of the day, unless you are buying milk…stay away from the rest of the sugary drinks.
The food and drinks that the child consumes during that day at the amusement park WILL make a difference in their mood, ability to self-regulate, and ability to cope with the sensory challenges at hand.

### Public Bathrooms

I can just hear it now…the dreaded HUGE public bathroom with VERY loud automatic flushing toilets and automatic hand dryers that sound like a plane taking off. And not just one…but 6-10 of each of these going on/off at different rates, unexpectedly! People rushing around in a hurry to get to the next ride, and sometimes screaming and crying babies on the changing table. I am in sensory overload just thinking about it.

Be prepared. Don't just rush your child in there without the right tools…noise cancelling headphones or earplugs, if needed. Carry your child into the bathroom providing a nice deep pressure hug. Don't rush her around and get into a tizzy like the rest of the people in the bathroom.

If at all possible, use the COMPANION RESTROOM or the FAMILY RESTROOM. This will cut down on a ton of this unnecessary sensory input.

### Enough is Enough

Staying in a hotel close to the amusement park can be your saving grace. Even though it may be a little more expensive to stay at a hotel on the grounds or very nearby, when your sensory kiddo has had enough…they have had enough. If you have more than one child with you, hopefully you also have an extra adult along with you. If so, then one parent can leave when your sensory kiddo is ready to go. Trying to push through is not the answer…it will only create a snowball effect, and the whole family will need a sensory retreat by the end of the day if you do so. Expect that you may need to leave early with your sensory kiddo.

# Water Parks

### Another Multi-Sensory Experience
Now there is an off season for the water parks in Florida, but it still may be a little chilly go in the off season. So for the most part, water parks are experienced in the summer only. My suggestion is to come early when they first open or at the end of the day. This can be very helpful in the overall experience.

I often "get on my soapbox" about how wonderful swimming is for a sensory kiddo, since it is an excellent way to get very powerful proprioception and also to develop body awareness and motor skills. The water park may be the exception to this rule.

A water park can be a real challenge for a sensory child as it is like an amusement park and the beach and the pool all combined into one challenging sensory environment. Sensory kiddos, especially sensory avoiders, are just as content at a nice calm neighborhood pool. They will likely not participate too much at the water park. You may find yourself separated from the rest of the family spending time in the calm and relaxing "basic pool" while everyone else if off doing the waterslides. Even the kiddo pool area may be too much splashing and screaming.

Now for a sensory seeker, a water park may sound like a great place, but there may be a safety issue. Since the child may get into her "sensory tunnel", the next thing you know, she may have run off to the wave pool and jumped into the deep end. A child needs direct supervision everywhere at the water park.


### The Rides
The tough part about the water park rides is that there usually is not a place for your belongings at the beginning of the ride. Typically there are lockers somewhere in the park instead. In this case, it is difficult to bring along some of your sensory tools while waiting in line. You cannot bring them on the ride due to the water factor, and there will not be a safe place to keep your belongings.

Water park rides are even more unpredictable than at an amusement park because, as we all know, on a water slide your body can get tossed and flipped in all directions, unlike when you are buckled into a basic amusement park ride. Also, usually at the end of a water ride there is the unexpected dump into a big pool of water, which can be very unpredictable, as well. Even for the sensory seekers this can be a very challenging thing.

Then you have the wave pool…this can be wonderful, but also a disaster. The wave pool is big, unpredictable, and powerful. Even when your child plays near the shore of the waves, it can be challenging, but also so tempting for the sensory seeker. Even if you bring your child out into the waves on a tube, be cautious and ready for the unexpected bump and flip of the tube from the people next to you going a little crazy. The wave pool seems to be such a popular and busy place all of the time.

### The Sun
The sun is draining and even more powerful when it reflects off the water. Be sure your sensory kiddo has a floppy hat and polarized sunglasses and spends plenty of time in the shade drinking a

ton of water. This component is tough on all of us, but even more challenging for a child faced with sensory challenges.

**Sensory Tools**
Here is a list of the essential tools for the water park…
- Putty swimmer's earplugs, not only for the sensation of the water, but to wear the entire time to limit auditory input
- Swimming goggles or a swimmer's mask
- Oral sensory tools and a Camelbak® water bottle with water only
- Floppy hat and polarized sunglasses
- Portable sensory retreat

**A Portable Sensory Retreat**
This was discussed in the previous section on amusement parks, so for the most part this information is repeated. But one of the essentials at the water park will need to be a stroller with a canopy or light weight blanket covering it for shade. The main components of the portable sensory retreat need to be:
- Cozy and squishy (lots of blankets and a stuffed animal or pillow)
- A blanket to cover the entire stroller to minimize all sensory input
- Something weighted if possible, such as a weighted lap pad or blanket
- Fidget toy and possibly a vibrating toy or vibrating pillow
- Oral sensory tools
- Crunchy and chewy snacks
- Earplugs or noise-cancelling headphones, MP3 player with soft calming music
- Possibly a floppy hat and sunglasses

You will want to use this sensory retreat often and throughout the day…not just when your child is in sensory overload. Be pro-active about it and use it as a place to re-group and help your sensory kiddo self-regulate. Use it between rides, anytime you are doing a lot of waiting, and whenever your child seems to need it or request it for a little down time.

**The Kiddo Pool**
The kiddie pool may be your home away from home with your little sensory seeker. And for your sensory avoider, it may be good in small doses. I would strongly recommend goggles or a mask even at a very young age, as well as swimmer's ear plugs. The feeling of the water splashing in the eyes and ears can be just the trigger to send your child into sensory overload. And we all know that the splashing is far from minimal at the water park in the kiddo pool.

**The Lazy River and Standard Pool**
My guess is with your sensory avoider you will find yourself spending most of your time in the lazy river (most water parks have one) and the standard, regular ol' pool. It is best to expect this and be prepared for this, because setting your expectations too high will only be a big disappointment and even perhaps frustrating for a parent.

This is also a great place for your sensory seeker to spend time…it is your best option for organizing and regulating sensory input. Your sensory seeker will need this being in an environment where sensory input abounds in a very multi-sensory and chaotic fashion.

### Accommodations for Special Needs

On **ASensoryLife.com** you will find links for various theme parks, as each one has their own process for accommodating special needs. I have also created a printable handout to use as documentation for this hidden disability.

🦋 **Safe Travels!**

For more information on all of the topics discussed in the handbook, please visit **ASensoryLife.com**!

**Enjoy the sensory journey!**

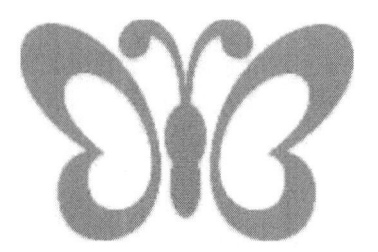

A page for your kiddo to scribble.

Printed in Great Britain
by Amazon.co.uk, Ltd.,
Marston Gate.